D0897562

A Phylogenetic Fantasy

A Phylogenetic Fantasy

Overview of the Transference Neuroses

SIGMUND FREUD

Edited and with an essay by
ILSE GRUBRICH-SIMITIS

Translated by
AXEL HOFFER AND PETER T. HOFFER

The Belknap Press of
Harvard University Press
Cambridge, Massachusetts
and London, England
1987

First published as *Übersicht der Übertragungsneurosen: Ein bisher unbekanntes Manuskript* (Frankfurt: S. Fischer Verlag, 1985)

Printed in the United States of America
10 9 8 7 6 5 4 3 2 1

This book is printed on acid-free paper, and its
binding materials have been chosen for strength and durability.

Library of Congress Cataloging-in-Publication Data

Freud, Sigmund, 1856–1939.
A phylogenetic fantasy.

Translation of: Übersicht der Übertragungsneurosen.
Bibliography: p.
1. Neuroses. 2. Transference (Psychology)
3. Psychoanalysis. I. Grubrich-Simitis, Ilse.
II. Title.
RC530.F73613 1987 616.85′2 86-26468
ISBN 0-674-66635-6

Design by Gwen Frankfeldt

Contents

Foreword
to the English-Language Edition

AXEL HOFFER AND PETER T. HOFFER

In 1983 Ilse Grubrich-Simitis came upon a previously unknown draft of Sigmund Freud's twelfth metapsychological paper. The unexpected discovery, described in her preface to this volume, provides a unique opportunity to reexamine from an evolutionary perspective Freud's thinking about the nature of man and of mental disorders. This occasion is of particular interest to students not only of psychoanalysis but also of the social sciences, humanities, and natural sciences. Psychoanalysis is built on the foundation of Freud's simple yet profound method of obtaining data about the dynamic functioning of the individual human mind by means of free association in the context of a psychoanalytic relationship (Kris, 1982). The psychoanalytic approach has been used in areas as diverse as mind-body relationships (psychology-biology), child development, and cultural anthropology, to mention only a few. The purview of psychoanalysis ranges from a microscopic focus on the psychic reality of one individual in a psychoanalytic treatment hour to a macroscopic focus on human nature in groups or societies, and even—as in this draft—in the prehistory of mankind.

One of the oldest controversies about—even within—the field of psychoanalysis is whether it is a biological science or a psychology independent of biology. The literature is replete with heated arguments on both sides. Sulloway (1979), for one, argues that Freud was *really* a biologist. Others (for instance Klein, 1976) assert that psychoanalysis is *really* a discipline of meaning and interpretation alone, divorced from biology, and therefore not a natural science. We feel that attempts to categorize Freud's distinctive method of investigation under one or another of the traditional disciplines are unnecessarily limiting. The uniqueness and value of Freud's discovery of a new method of investigation—that of free association—lies in the unfettered freedom to explore human differences, conflicts, and dilemmas. We believe that psychoanalysis should not be categorized as belonging either to the natural sciences (the *Naturwissenschaften*) or to the humanities (the *Geisteswissenschaften*) alone, but to both. Freud's overview is an example of the way in which the inextricable theoretical bonds between psychology and biology provide fertile fields for new investigations leading to new points of view.

The discovery and identification of a draft of Freud's synthesis of the transference neuroses, the fair copy of which Freud subsequently destroyed, have aroused great interest. The paper itself is part of an intense correspondence between Freud and his colleague Sándor Ferenczi during the dark days early in World War I. Such a manuscript is like an archaeological discovery, perhaps hiding buried within it a key to deeper understanding—in this case, of Freud's earlier and later writings.

Grubrich-Simitis has attempted to present Freud's work in unmodified form exactly as she found it, leaving primarily to the reader the interpretation of its possible meanings and ultimate significance. In her essay, "Metapsychology and Metabiology," she writes on the place of the phylogenetic fantasy in Freud's life and work and in the history of science. She traces the context of the unearthed draft, saving evaluative and analytical comments for the third part of the essay.

What is the overview actually about? None of Freud's metapsychological papers is easy to read, and this one is no exception. To help orient the reader, we therefore attempt in this Foreword to highlight the major themes and transition points elaborated in Grubrich-Simitis' essay.

Freud wrote a draft of his nearly completed twelfth metapsychological paper in the form of a letter to Ferenczi, inviting his knowledgeable colleague's critical response. The draft has two distinct parts, the first of which utilizes a staccato, shorthand style in which Freud presents the characteristics of the three transference neuroses (anxiety hysteria, conversion hysteria, and obsessional neurosis). He compares and contrasts six factors in these three disorders: repression, anticathexis, substitutive- and symptom-formation, relation to the sexual function, regression, and disposition.

Freud's discussion of these mechanisms is entirely consistent with his published metapsychological papers in that he is working within his topographic theory based on the systems unconscious, preconscious, and conscious. He has yet to develop his structural theory based on conflict within and among three agencies (ego, id, and super-ego), which many psychoanalysts feel serves more as an addition to than as a replacement for the earlier topographic theory. As Grubrich-Simitis elaborates in her essay later in this volume, Freud was working within his first theory of anxiety (sometimes called his toxicological theory), based on "dammed-up libido" as a "cause" of symptoms and illness. Only later, with *Inhibitions, Symptoms and Anxiety* (1926d [1925]),[1] did he fully articulate his second theory of anxiety, in which anxiety served a "signal" function to mobilize the ego's defense mechanisms.

Similarly, Freud's dual-instinct theory evolved after the overview was written from a theory based on the polarity between sexual instincts and ego- (self-preservative) instincts to one based on the polarity between life (sexual) instincts and death (aggressive) instincts. This paper may be seen, then, as a transitional document immediately preceding Freud's major theoretical shifts toward the end of the war. After World War I, when publication of this and the six other lost papers became feasible, Freud might have felt he had left this work far behind in his new theoretical advances.

Our translation of this work has been called "A Phylogenetic Fantasy" because it is in this area that Freud's contribution is new. His own title, "Overview of the Transference Neuroses," is actually a misnomer. Freud undoubtedly would have changed it had he published the paper, because he not only covers the transference neuroses (anxiety, conversion hysteria, and obsessional neurosis) but, with equal importance, brings in the narcissistic neuroses (dementia praecox,[2] paranoia, and melancholia-mania). The crucial points hinge on the detailed comparisons between the way people with transference neuroses are able to establish and maintain relationships, and the way those with narcissistic neuroses have difficulty maintaining a firm grasp on their interpersonal relationships and on reality.

The first hint of the importance of this comparison occurs early in the draft. Freud says on the opening page (edited form of the manuscript), "Will hear that in the next group repression has a different topography; it then becomes extended to the concept of splitting."

1. For an explanation of the system of citation used throughout, see the note at the beginning of the References.

2. Emil Kraepelin's term *dementia praecox* would today, following Eugen Bleuler's terminology, become *schizophrenia*.

The essential link between the first part of the paper and the second lies in Freud's discussion of the sixth factor, disposition. Here he makes the transition, believing that when constitutional factors come into consideration "acquisition [is] not eliminated thereby; it only moves into still earlier prehistory, because one can justifiably claim that the inherited dispositions are residues of the acquisition of our ancestors" (p. 10). Having paved the way for the importance of the "phylogenetic disposition," he adds:

> The most important distinguishing characteristic of the transference neuroses could not be acknowledged in this overview anyway, because it is not striking when they are compared with one another and would only become evident by contrast when the narcissistic neuroses are brought in. With this widening of the horizon ⟨the⟩[3] relation of ego to object would move [into the] foreground, and the holding onto the object would turn out to be ⟨the⟩ common distinguishing feature. (pp. 10–11)

The final introductory comments are crucial to following the thrust of Freud's argument, as we shall see.

> We must ascribe a different development to the sexual strivings of man than to the ego-strivings. The reason ⟨is⟩ essentially that the former can be satisfied autoerotically for quite a while, whereas ego-strivings from the beginning are directed at object and thereby at reality. (p. 11)

Thus, Freud organizes his conceptualization of the transference neuroses around anxiety and sexuality, and his conceptualization of the narcissistic neuroses around the loss of the object.

The second section of the draft, unlike the first, is written in complete sentences. Freud himself referred to this second part as his "phylogenetic fantasy," a term that highlights the original and creative aspects of the work. In a creative leap of imagination he brings together for the first time not just the customary two (ontogeny recapitulates phylogeny) developmental sequences, but rather three:

1. The development of the individual (ontogeny);
2. The development of the species (phylogeny);
3. The developmental sequence of the age of onset of the two groups of mental disorders—first, the transference neuroses (anxiety hysteria, conversion hysteria, and obsessional neurosis) and second, the narcissistic neuroses (dementia praecox, paranoia, and melancholia-mania).

3. Angle brackets, ⟨ ⟩, signify a translators' addition.

In attempting to group specific mental disorders according to the typical age of onset, Freud explores the possibility that there is a correlation between mental disorders and the history of the adaptations required for the survival of mankind. The first threat was the one posed by the geologic development of the earth, the Ice Age; the second threat came from the relation of the sons to the father before and after the murder of the patriarch.

In what we might consider the first generation of sons, therefore, the threats to survival during the Ice Age correlate with the climatic changes and the development of human hordes under the primal father. As is shown in Grubrich-Simitis' essay, the characteristics of the three transference neuroses are understood as adaptive initially to privations caused by changes in climate and subsequently to the growing threats of castration by the father.

For the second generation of sons the organizing principle of the next three phases of the development of society, after the Ice Age, lies in the actuality of the (older) sons' castration by the jealous and vengeful patriarch and his ultimate murder by the sons. The three narcissistic neuroses thus belong to the second generation of sons. Freud's postulate of a link between the impact on the sons of the primal father's growing tyranny and the disorder of dementia praecox is very difficult to follow. He connects the "historical" event of the sons' castration with the symptoms of dementia praecox:

> We may imagine the effect of castration in that primeval time as an extinguishing of the libido and a standstill in individual development. Such a state . . . leads to giving up every love-object, degeneration of all sublimations, and return to autoerotism. The youthful individual behaves as though he had undergone castration. In fact, self-castrations are not uncommon with this disorder. (p. 17)

In Freud's scheme the trauma of castration by the father somehow leads to impairment of the dementia praecox patient's capacity for holding onto object relationships. Whether that incapacity is also related to the subsequent murder of the father is unclear. In the second phase, the sons flee the brutal father and gather in groups where paranoia serves as a presumably adaptive defense against homosexuality. Finally, in the third phase, the brothers overpower and kill the primal father. They feel triumphant about his death, then mourn him because they still revere him as a model. Melancholia-mania thus is the modern precipitate of the alternating experiences of the loss of the father and narcissistic identification with him. We can now see how in his phylogenetic fantasy Freud modifies and expands the reasoning he began in *Totem and Taboo* (1912–13).

Freud's organization and sequences may be particularly difficult for the reader to follow because we are unaccustomed to thinking of anxiety and hysteria as earlier or more primitive than dementia praecox. Freud, of course, wrote about this paradoxical inversion of the developmental sequences of the sexual and the ego-instincts, but it sounds odd to modern ears. It may be helpful to keep in mind that his argument here is based on the premise that sexual instincts have an earlier (more purely biological) and entirely different development than the ego- (self-preservative) instincts. Freud also took as a premise for his series that narcissistic neuroses do not occur in childhood, an assumption not supported by present-day work with children.

In the relevant Freud-Ferenczi correspondence, published here for the first time, the interest of both men in Lamarckian concepts is explicitly discussed and documented. Freud in the phylogenetic fantasy extends his belief in the inheritance of acquired characteristics as far as it will go. Grubrich-Simitis, in her essay, discusses the reasons for Freud's insistence on the reality of the inheritance of past experience. She suggests that Freud felt that the intensity of the castration/murder complex in each generation can only be explained by such a hereditary transmission from one generation to the next.

Freud ultimately concludes that each individual contains somewhere within himself or herself the history of all mankind; further, that mental illness can usefully be understood as a vestige of responses once necessary and highly adaptive to the exigencies of each era. Accordingly, mental illness can be understood as a set of formerly adaptive responses that have become maladaptive as the climatic and sociological threats to the survival of mankind have changed.

Beyond the historical interest of this document with its outdated aspects, there is an unambiguous link to modern psychoanalysis in Freud's emphasis on the theme of adaptation, in the development of both the individual and mankind. It is important to understand that what is involved is adaptation in a broad, psychoanalytic sense, not (as it has been so frequently misunderstood in the past) adaptation in the sense of conformity to society's expectations. Contemporary psychoanalysts study in increasingly complex ways the adaptation of the individual and of groups to intrapsychic and interpersonal conflict. For example, psychoanalysts today have made significant advances in appreciating the priority of issues of safety—the perception of a threat to psychological survival—in the analytic setting (see for example Sandler, 1960; Shafer, 1983; Modell, 1984). They have a more sophisticated understanding of the ways in which conflicts arising (1) from drives and defenses against them, (2) from conflicting drives (Kris, 1984), and (3) as a result of specific affective states trigger unconscious and conscious defense mechanisms. These mechanisms are always adaptive for internal psychic reality and homeostasis, but often are maladaptive in terms of relationships and external reality. The concerns of psychoanalysts in attempting to understand human beings range from the microscopic view of an anxious moment in an analytic hour to cosmic issues raised by the threat of nuclear annihilation. Adaptation to perceived danger and the maladaptive aspects of "too much" adaptation for the individual and society remain vital psychoanalytic issues.

No new translation of Freud can be attempted without taking into account the recent critiques by Mahoney (1982, 1984), Ornston (1982, 1985), Bettelheim (1983), and others of James Strachey's *Standard Edition of the Complete Psychological Works of Sigmund Freud*. Malcolm Pines (1985) and the Publications Committee of the Institute of Psychoanalysis (London), representing the International Library of Psychoanalysis, are currently giving careful thought to the complex question of whether the *Standard Edition* should be revised or whether a completely new translation of Freud should be undertaken.

For a number of reasons we have chosen to translate this draft in a way that does not involve any significant new renderings which would conflict with the conventions established by Strachey in his translation of the metapsychology papers published in the *Standard Edition*. We hope that the reader will thereby find it easier to compare this paper with and integrate it into the existing corpus of Freud's metapsychological writings. In addition to following Strachey, we have used the publication of the Glossary Committee (Jones, 1924) and Alix Strachey's *Vocabulary* (1943) to help us with some of the technical terms.

Our translation of the draft of the twelfth metapsychological paper has led us to a better appreciation of the challenges faced by A. A. Brill, Anna Freud, Ernest Jones, John Rickman, Joan Riviere, James and Alix Strachey, Alan Tyson, and others in trying to render Freud's precise scientific writing into the English language with minimal loss of meaning, context, and style. We are brothers from a German-speaking background (Czechoslovakia), educated in the United States. Peter Hoffer, a professor of German, has played the primary role in the actual translation; Axel Hoffer, a practicing psychoanalyst and teacher, is principally responsible for this Foreword—but in all senses the work has been a collaborative effort.

In our translation of both the Freud draft and the Grubrich-Simitis essay, we have refrained insofar as possible from imposing our interpretations on the material. Particularly in the first half of the paper, we have retained the shorthand style of the draft, sacrificing ease of understanding to capture the flavor—and the ambiguity—of Freud's writing. In general, we have favored a literal translation, which may at times have a Germanic tone, in order to be more faithful to the original.

We are deeply appreciative of the helpful criticism and encouragement provided by Otto Hoffer, Anton O. Kris, Arnold H. Modell, Ana-Maria Rizzuto, Angela von der Lippe, and Vivian Wheeler. We thank Arthur Rosenthal, director of Harvard University Press, for his steadfast support and for his commitment to this project. And we are grateful to Ilse Grubrich-Simitis for her invaluable and most generous assistance with the translation. She not only made available to us her remarkable command of the English language, but also shared her profound insight into Freud's language and thought.

September 1986

Preface

to the Original Edition

ILSE GRUBRICH-SIMITIS

From November 1914 until the summer of 1915 Sigmund Freud worked on a series of papers that he originally intended to publish in book form under the title *Zur Vorbereitung einer Metapsychologie* (Preliminaries to a metapsychology). In a note to one of the texts, "A Metapsychological Supplement to the Theory of Dreams" (1917d [1915]), which appeared in 1917, he stated their purpose: "The intention of the series is to clarify and carry deeper the theoretical assumptions on which a psycho-analytic system could be founded" (p. 222). Also belonging to this series and not published until 1917 is "Mourning and Melancholia" (1917e [1915]). By contrast, three other pieces written in the first months of the war year 1915 were published that same year in successive issues of the *Internationale Zeitschrift für ärztliche Psychoanalyse* (vol. 3, nos. 2–5). These three papers are the classic basic writings of psychoanalysis—"Instincts and Their Vicissitudes" (1915c), "Repression" (1915d), and "The Unconscious" (1915e). James Strachey (1957b, p. 161) has designated the five metapsychological papers as perhaps Freud's most important theoretical works.

From his correspondence we know that, in addition to the five texts mentioned, Freud had by mid-1915 more or less completed seven other metapsychological studies, which were supposed to round off the series for a book of twelve chapters.[1] The book was never published, however. Because the seven later manuscripts disappeared without a trace, it is assumed that Freud subsequently destroyed them. "It is difficult," as Strachey wrote, "to exaggerate our loss from the disappearance of these

1. This was reconstructed by Ernest Jones (1955, pp. 185–186). In the course of writing his Freud biography, he was the first to see Freud's correspondence, which at that time was largely unpublished.

papers. There was a unique conjunction of favourable factors at the time at which Freud wrote them. His previous major theoretical work (the seventh chapter of the *Interpretation of Dreams* [1900a]) had been written fifteen years before, at a relatively early stage of his psychological studies. Now, however, he had some twenty-five years of psycho-analytic experience behind him on which to base his theoretical constructions, while he remained at the summit of his intellectual powers" (1957a, p. 106).

Last year in London—in connection with preparations for the forthcoming publication of the correspondence between Freud and his Hungarian student and colleague, Sándor Ferenczi—I was looking through an old trunk of papers and other documents that had been given to the Hungarian-born psychoanalyst Michael Balint by his teacher and friend, Ferenczi. I came upon a manuscript in Freud's handwriting which from its title and content I could not connect with any of his published works. With the help of a brief letter Freud had written on the back of the last page, I soon realized what the manuscript was: the draft[2] of the lost twelfth metapsychological paper. The letter reads:[3]

7/28/15

Dear friend,

I am sending you herewith the draft of the XII [paper], which will certainly interest you. You can throw it away or keep it. The fair copy follows it sentence for sentence, deviating from it only slightly. Pages 21–23 have been added since your letter, which I had waited for. Fortunately, I had anticipated your excellent criticism.[4]

2. The discovery of this manuscript incidentally permits modification of my own observations (1977, p. 40) about Freud's writing process in the facsimile edition of his essay "The Theme of the Three Caskets"—namely, that although he was accustomed to writing out the final version of his manuscripts immediately, he made only few corrections at any one time. These comments were based on information from Freud's daughter Anna and on perusal of the manuscripts of Freud's works that have been preserved since 1914. These manuscripts are always fair copies. Possibly the majority of them existed in drafts, which Freud did not save. In the end he would not have preserved the recently discovered draft; on the contrary, in the accompanying letter he left it up to Ferenczi to throw the manuscript away or to keep it. Because Ferenczi kept it, we now know that Freud wrote drafts and that, as the second part shows, these could take almost final form and did not contain many corrections.

3. The facsimile appears on p. 71. It has been transcribed in accordance with the rules applied to the manuscript as a whole, which are explained in the Note on the Edited Version.

4. For details see pp. 80–81.

I will take a break now, before I finally work out Cs. [consciousness] and anxiety. I am suffering greatly from Karlsbad [intestinal] ailments.

Warm regards,

Your Freud

The letter makes it possible to identify the manuscript with certainty.[5] Freud corresponded regularly with Ferenczi in 1915 about his metapsychology project; furthermore, from this letter and other correspondence we can infer the themes of the seven lost chapters: among them consciousness, anxiety/anxiety hysteria (the work on both these texts is expressly mentioned in the letter above), conversion hysteria, obsessional neurosis—as well as, in fact, a synthesis of the transference neuroses. And now, in the draft overview, we obtain firsthand knowledge of the content of this synthesis.

I should like to thank Ingeborg Meyer-Palmedo for her indefatigable support in the publication of this work, particularly for her careful preparation of the transcription, which is totally faithful to the original. Enid Balint of London made it possible to copy the original manuscript and gave much invaluable help.

November 1984

5. Additional arguments appear on pp. 78ff.

Overview of the Transference Neuroses

SIGMUND FREUD

The Edited Version

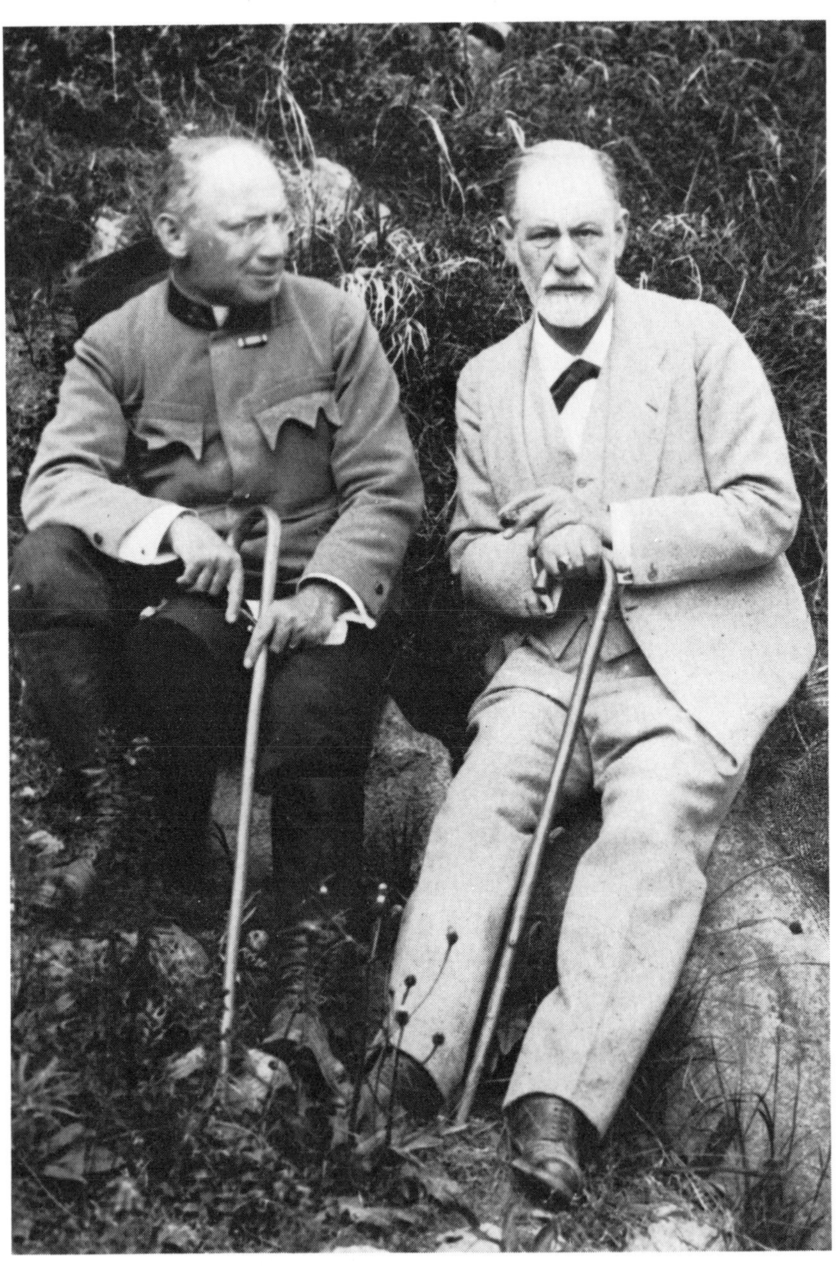

Sándor Ferenczi and Sigmund Freud during a vacation in the Tatra Mountains of Czechoslovakia in the summer of 1917.

Note on the Edited Version

As both facsimile and literal transcription show, Freud's manuscript contains a plethora of abbreviations, especially of word endings. In the interest of readability these have been silently expanded in this version of the draft. Where this could not be done with certainty, my additions have been indicated by square brackets, [ ]; those of the translators by angle brackets, ⟨ ⟩. The only abbreviations that have been retained are those especially characteristic of Freud, such as "Ucs." (unconscious), "Pcs." (preconscious), "Cs." (conscious), "ΨA" (psychoanalysis).

On the other hand, the shorthand character of the original, especially in the systematic first part, ought not be obliterated by editorial amplifications; this is after all only a draft, not the fair copy. In only a very few places have I attempted to facilitate understanding by adding words. These are without exception flagged with square brackets, in part because I have not always been sure that they are correct. Orthography and punctuation have been silently aligned with modern usage. Editorial footnotes call attention to certain peculiarities of the original, so that the reader can locate them in the facsimile without undue difficulty.

I.G.-S.

XII Overview of the Transference Neuroses

Preliminaries

After detailed investigation, attempt to summarize characteristics, distinguishing from others, comparative survey of the individual factors. Factors are repression, anticathexis,[1] substitutive- and symptom-formation, relation to the sexual function, regression, disposition. Restriction to the three types: anxiety hysteria, conversion hysteria, and obsessional neurosis.

(a) *Repression* takes place in all three at the border of the system Ucs. and Pcs., consists in the withdrawal or renunciation [of the] Pcs. cathexis, is secured by means of a kind of anticathexis. In later stages of obsessional neurosis displaces itself to the border between Pcs. and Cs.

Will hear that in the next group[2] repression has a different topography; it then becomes extended to the concept of splitting.

Topographical point of view should not be overestimated in the sense that perhaps all interchange between both systems is interrupted by it. It thus becomes more important at which elements this barrier is introduced.

Success and completeness are related insofar as failure necessitates further efforts. Success varies with the three neuroses and in their individual stages.

Least success with anxiety hysteria, is confined to the fact that no Pcs. (and Cs.) representative comes about. Later, that instead of the offensive

1. Originally, *Gegenbesetzung* (anticathexis) was the third item in this sequence; by means of an insertion line Freud moved the word to the second position. See facsimile p. 1, ll. 6–7.

2. Probably meant here are the psychoses (or, in Freud's usage, the narcissistic neuroses), referred to in the second part of the draft but admittedly not described in more detail in relation to the specific processes of defense. See pp. 233–235 of "A Metapsychological Supplement to the Theory of Dreams" (1917d [1915]).

⟨one⟩, a substitutive [idea] becomes Pcs. and Cs. Finally, in the formation of phobias it achieves its aim, in inhibiting the affect of unpleasure by means of great renunciation, extensive attempt at flight. Intent of repression is always avoidance of unpleasure. Fate of the representative is only a sign of the process. The apparent[3] separation into idea and affect (representative and quantitative factor) of the process to be defended against results from the very fact that repression consists in the renunciation of the word-presentation, thus from [the] topographical character of the repression.

In obsessional neurosis success is at first complete but not lasting. Process still less complete. After first successful phase it continues through two additional ones, the first of which (secondary repression[:][4] formation of the obsessional idea, struggle against obsessional idea) satisfies itself, as [in] anxiety hysteria, with substitution of the representative, [the] later [phase] (tertiary [repression]) produces renunciations and restriction[s] that correspond to the phobia, but in contrast operates by logical means.

In contradistinction to this, success of conversion hysteria is from the outset[5] complete, but at the cost of strong substitutive formation. Process of the individual repression more complete.

(b) *Anticathexis*[6]

In anxiety hysteria, missing at first[,] pure attempt at flight, then throws itself at substitutive idea and, especially in third phase, at its surroundings, in order from there to secure control of the release of unpleasure, as[7] watchfulness, attentiveness. Represents the portion of the Pcs. [cathexis]; in other words, the expenditure that neurosis costs.

In obsessional neurosis, where from the outset it has to do with defense against an ambivalent instinct, it provides for the first successful repression, then achieves reaction-formation thanks to the ambivalence, then in

3. At this point the manuscript (p. 2) is hard to decipher. The words *deskriptiv statt syst[ematisch]* (descriptive instead of syst[ematic]) have been added between ll. 3 and 4, a formulation that Freud also uses in "The Unconscious" (1915e, p. 172).

4. The further items up to the closing parenthesis are located in the manuscript (p. 2) at the end of the section, just before (b); evidently added afterward, they were clearly transposed to the indicated position by means of a line.

5. In the manuscript (p. 2, l. 20) there is an erroneous repetition of *ein* instead of *an*.

6. Here in the manuscript (p. 2, l. 24) is written, and crossed out, *Ersatz u Symptombildg.* (substitutive- and symptom-formation). Apparently Freud decided at this point in the writing to treat anticathexis before substitutive- and symptom-formation. See the corresponding inversion in the series at the beginning of the paper.

7. This word cannot be deciphered with certainty. See p. 2, l. 30 of the facsimile.

the tertiary phase results in the attentiveness that characterizes the obsessional idea, and does the logical work. Thus, second and third phase just as in anxiety hysteria. Difference in first phase, where [the anticathexis] in anxiety hysteria accomplishes nothing, in obsessional neurosis everything.

Always it secures for repression [the] corre[sponding] portion of the Pcs. In [conversion] hysteria, successful[8] character is made possible by the fact that anticathexis seeks from the outset to join with instinctual cathexis and reaches a compromise with it, makes selective determination of representative.

(c) *Substitutive- and Symptom-Formation*

Corresponds to the return [of the] repressed, failure of repression. [Both can be] separated for a while, later [the substitutive-formation] fuses with it [the symptom-formation].

Most complete in the case of conversion hysteria: substitute = symptom, nothing further to be separated.

Likewise in anxiety hysteria, substitutive-formation makes possible the first return of the repressed.

In obsessional neurosis [substitutive] separates sharply [from symptom-formation] in that first substitutive-formation is delivered from the repressing by means of anticathexis and is not counted among symptoms. Whereas [the] later symptoms of obsessional neurosis are often predominantly return of the repressed; role of the repressing in them smaller.

Symptom-formation, where our investigation starts, always coincides with return of the repressed and occurs with the aid of regression and the disposing fixations. A general law states that the regression goes back to the fixation and from there return of the repressed asserts itself.

(d) *Relation to the Sexual Function*

What remains constant here is that repressed instinctual impulse is always a libidinal one, belonging to sexual life, whereas repression proceeds from the ego out of various motives, which can be summed up as a not-being-able-to (because of excessive strength) or a not-wanting-to. The latter goes back to incompatibility with the ego-ideals or to other kinds of feared injury to the ego. The not-being-able-to also corresponds to an injury.

This fundamental fact is clouded by two considerations. First, it often seems as though repression is aroused by conflict between two impulses,

8. Nor can this word be deciphered with certainty. See p. 3, l. 6 of the facsimile.

both [of which] are libidinal. This is resolved by considering that one of them is ego-syntonic and in the conflict can enlist the aid of the repression that emanates from the ego. Second, by virtue of the fact that not only libidinal but also ego-strivings are encountered among the repressed, especially frequent and distinct with longer duration and more advanced development of the neurosis. [The] latter comes about in such a way that the repressed libidinal impulse seeks to assert itself in a roundabout way by means of an ego-striving to which it has lent a component, transfers energy to it, and now pulls this [ego-striving] along into repression, which can occur on a large scale. Nothing in the general validity of the former statement is thereby altered. Understandable requirement that one gather insights from the beginning stages of the neuroses.

⟨It is⟩ evident in hysteria and obsessional neurosis that repression directs itself toward the[9] sexual function in definitive form, in which it[10] represents reproductive urge. Most distinct again in conversion hysteria, because without complications, in obsessional neurosis first regression. Meanwhile not exaggerate this connection, for instance, not assume that repression only goes into effect with this stage of the libido. On the contrary, it is precisely obsessional neurosis that shows that repression ⟨is a⟩ general process, not libidinally dependent, because here ⟨it is⟩ directed against preliminary stage. Likewise in development, that repression is also taken up against perverse impulses. Question: Why does repression succeed here, not elsewhere? In nature libidinal strivings very capable of representation, so that with repression of the normal, the perverse are strengthened, and vice versa. Repression has no relation to the sexual function other than to strive for its defense, like regression and other instinctual vicissitudes.

In anxiety hysteria the relation to the sexual function is less distinct, for reasons that have become apparent in the treatment of anxiety. Seems that anxiety hysteria encompasses those cases in which demands of sexual instinct [are] defended against as too great, like danger. No special condition from libido organization.

9. *Das* ⟨the neuter definite article in German⟩ was originally written at this point (perhaps Freud wanted to write *das Sexualleben*); the word is crossed out and replaced with *die* ⟨the feminine article, because the German word for sexual function is feminine⟩. See p. 4, l. 33 of the facsimile.

10. The original (p. 4, l. 34) has *es* ⟨the neuter pronoun⟩. See note 9.

(e) *Regression*

The most interesting factor and instinctual vicissitude. No occasion to divine it from anxiety hysteria. Could say that [it] does not enter into consideration here, perhaps because every later anxiety hysteria so clearly regresses to an infantile one (the typical disposition of neurosis), and this latter one appears so early in life. On the other hand, both of the other [transference neuroses] ⟨are the⟩ most beautiful examples of regression, but in each it plays a different role in structure of the neurosis. In conversion hysteria it is a strong ego regression, return to phase without separation of Pcs. and Ucs., thus without speech and censorship. Regression, however, serves symptom-formation and return of the repressed. The instinctual impulse that [is] not accepted by the current ego returns to an earlier one, from which it finds discharge, naturally in another manner. That it virtually comes to a kind of libido regression in the process ⟨has⟩ already ⟨been⟩ mentioned. It is different in obsessional neurosis. The regression is a libido regression, does not serve the return [of the repressed], but rather repression, and is made possible by a strong constitutional fixation or incomplete development. In fact, here the first step of defense is assigned to regression, where it is more a case of regression than to inhibition of development,[11] and the regressive libidinal organization is only subsequently subjected to a typical repression—which, however, remains unsuccessful. A piece of ego regression is forced upon [the] ego by the libido or is given in the incomplete development of the ego, which here is connected to libido phase. (Separation of ambivalences.)

(f) [*Disposition*]

Behind regression are hidden the problems of fixation and disposition. Regression, one can say in general, goes all the way back to a fixation point, in either ego or libido development, and it represents the disposition.[12] This is thus the most decisive factor, the one that mediates the decision concerning [the] choice of neurosis. ⟨It is⟩ worthwhile, therefore, to stay with it. Fixation comes about through ⟨a⟩ phase of development that was too strongly pronounced or has perhaps persisted too long to pass over into the next without residue. ⟨It⟩ would be best if [one] did not

11. This obscure clause seems to make more sense by positioning its word elements differently: "where it is a case of more than [a] regression to [an] inhibition of development."

12. In "The Disposition to Obsessional Neurosis" (1913i, p. 318) Freud declares plainly, "Thus our dispositions are inhibitions in development."

demand [a] clearer idea of what, in what changes, fixation consists. But say something about ⟨its⟩ origin. The possibility exists as well that such fixation is brought along in pure form and that it [is] also produced by early impressions and, in the end, that both factors work together. All the more since one can claim that both kinds of elements are actually ubiquitous, inasmuch as, [on the one hand,] all dispositions are constitutionally present in the child and, on the other hand, the operative impressions are allotted to large numbers of children in like manner. Is thus a case of more or less, and an effective coincidence. Because no one is inclined to dispute constitutional factors, it devolves upon ΨA to represent forcefully the interests of early infantile acquisitions. In obsessional neurosis, by the way, the constitutional factor is admittedly far more clearly recognized than is the accidental in conversion hysteria. Detailed assessment still doubtful.

When the constitutional factor of fixation comes into consideration, acquisition [is] not eliminated thereby; it only moves into still earlier prehistory, because one can justifiably claim that the inherited dispositions are residues of the acquisition of our ancestors. With this one runs into ⟨the⟩ problem of the phylogenetic disposition behind the individual or ontogenetic, and should find no contradiction[13] if the individual adds new dispositions from his own experience to his inherited disposition ⟨acquired⟩ on the basis of earlier experience. Why should the process that creates disposition on the basis of experience cease precisely at the individual whose neurosis one is investigating? Or ⟨why should⟩ this [individual] create [a] disposition for his progeny but not be able to acquire it for himself? Seems rather ⟨to be⟩ necessary complement.

How much the phylogenetic disposition can contribute to the[14] understanding of the neuroses cannot yet be estimated. Part of it would also be that consideration goes beyond narrow field of the transference neuroses. The most important distinguishing characteristic of the transference neuroses could not be acknowledged in this overview anyway, because it is not striking when they are compared with one another and would only become evident by contrast when the narcissistic neuroses are brought

13. In the middle of the word (p. 7, l. 32) Freud first wrote "t" instead of "p," perhaps in the direction of "resistance" ⟨*Widerstand*, instead of *Widerspruch* (contradiction), which appears in the manuscript⟩, and then corrected himself.

14. In the manuscript (p. 8, l. 9), *das* (the) is written, instead of *zum* (to the).

in.[15] With this widening of the horizon ⟨the⟩ relation of ego to object would move [into the] foreground, and the holding onto the object would turn out to be ⟨the⟩ common distinguishing feature. Certain preliminaries permitted here.

Hope the reader, who for no reason other than boredom over many sections has noticed how everything has been built on very careful and arduous observation, will be patient if once in a while criticism retreats in the face of fantasy and unconfirmed things are presented, merely because they are stimulating and open up distant vistas.

It is still legitimate to assume that the neuroses must also bear witness to the history of the mental development of mankind. Now I believe I have shown in ⟨the⟩ paper ("On Two Principles")[16] that we must ascribe a different development to the sexual strivings of man than to the ego-strivings. The reason ⟨is⟩ essentially that the former can be satisfied auto-erotically for quite a while, whereas ego-strivings from the beginning are directed at object and thereby at reality. [As for] the development of[17] human sexual life, we believe we have learned to understand it in broad outline (*Three Essays on the Theory of Sexuality* [1905d]). That of the human ego, that is, of the functions of self-preservation and the formations derived from them, is more difficult to fathom. I know only the single attempt of Ferenczi,[18] who makes use of ψα experiences for this purpose. Our task would naturally be much easier if the developmental history of the ego were given to us somewhere else of understanding the neuroses, instead of our having to proceed in the opposite direction.[19] One thereby gets the impression that the developmental history of the libido recapitulates a much older piece of the [phylogenetic] development than that of the

15. Two crossed-out sentence fragments follow in the manuscript (p. 8, ll. 18–20): *Er liegt in der Festhaltung des Objekts. Verhältnis des Ich zum Objekt.* (It lies in the holding onto the object. Relation of the ego to the object.)

16. "Formulations on the Two Principles of Mental Functioning" (1911b).

17. In the manuscript (p. 9, l. 10), *der* ⟨the genitive case, feminine form of the definite article, instead of the masculine *des*⟩; Freud probably first intended to write *der menschlichen Sexualität* (of human sexuality) ⟨which is feminine⟩.

18. Sándor Ferenczi (1913).

19. This passage probably means, "Our task of understanding the neuroses would naturally be much easier if the developmental history of the ego were given to us somewhere else instead of our having to proceed in the opposite direction [that is, inferring the developmental history of the ego from the investigation of the neuroses]." Freud possibly added the phrase *die Neurosen zu verstehen* (of understanding the neuroses) in the continuing text afterward, as was customary for him, but forgot to insert an arrow.

ego; the former perhaps recapitulates conditions of the phylum of vertebrates, whereas the latter is dependent on the history of the human race. Now there exists a series to which one can attach various far-reaching ideas. It originates when one arranges the Ψ neuroses (not the transference neuroses alone) according to the[20] point in time at which they customarily appear in the life of the individual. Then anxiety hysteria, almost without precondition, is the earliest [neurosis], closely followed by conversion hysteria (from about the fourth year); somewhat later in prepuberty (9–10) obsessional neurosis appears in children. The narcissistic neuroses are absent in childhood. Of these, dementia praecox in classic form is [an] illness of the puberty years, paranoia approaches the mature years, and melancholia-mania the same time period, otherwise not specifiable.

The series is thus:

anxiety hysteria — conversion hysteria — obsessional neurosis — dementia praecox — paranoia — melancholia-mania.

The fixation dispositions of these disorders also appear to produce a series, which runs in the opposite direction, however,[21] especially when one takes libidinal dispositions into consideration. The result would thus be that the later the neurosis appears, the earlier the phase of the libido to which it must regress. But this only holds true in general terms. Undoubtedly conversion hysteria is directed against primacy of the genitals, obsessional neurosis against the sadistic preliminary stage, all three transference neuroses against complete development of the libido. The narcissistic neuroses, however, go back to phases before the finding of object; dementia praecox regresses as far as auto-erotism; paranoia as far as narcissistic homosexual object-choice; melancholia is based on narcissistic identification with the object. The differences lie in the fact that dementia unquestionably appears earlier than paranoia, although its libidinal disposition extends farther back, and that melancholia-mania permit⟨s⟩ no certain ranking with respect to time. One can therefore not maintain that the time sequence of the Ψneuroses, which certainly exists, was determined solely by the development of the libido. To the extent that this is the case, one

20. The manuscript (p. 9, l. 35) reads *der* ⟨the dative case of the feminine definite article⟩, because Freud first wrote *nach der Zeit* (after the time), then added *punkt* (point) ⟨which makes the word masculine⟩, and neglected to change the article accordingly.

21. At this point in the manuscript (p. 10, l. 15) the word *Deutlich* (Clearly) is crossed out.

would emphasize the inverse relationship between the two. It is also known that with advancing age hysteria or obsessional neurosis can turn into dementia; the opposite never occurs.

One can set up another phylogenetic series, however, which is really concurrent with the time sequence of the neuroses. Only in doing so, one must go far afield and allow some hypothetical intermediate link.

Dr. Wittels[22] first expressed the idea that the primal human animal passed its existence in a thoroughly rich milieu that satisfied all needs, echoes of which we have retained in the myth of the primeval paradise. There it may have overcome the periodicity of the libido, which is still connected with mammals. Ferenczi,[23] in the aforementioned thoughtful paper, then expressed the idea that the subsequent development of this primal human took place under the influence of the geological fate of the earth, and that the exigencies of the Ice Age[24] in particular gave it the stimulus for the development of civilization. After all, it is generally conceded that the human race already existed at the time of the Ice Age and experienced its effects.

If we pursue Ferenczi's idea, the temptation is very great to recognize[25] in the three dispositions to anxiety hysteria, conversion hysteria, and obsessional neurosis regressions to phases that the whole human race had to go through at some time from the beginning to the end of the Ice Age, so that at that time all human beings were the way only some of them are today, by virtue of their hereditary tendency and by means of new acquisition. The pictures naturally cannot coincide completely, because neurosis contains more than what regression brings with it. It is also the expression of the struggle against this regression and a compromise between the primevally old and the demands of the culturally new. This difference will have to be most strongly pronounced in obsessional neurosis, which like no other stands under the sign of inner conflict. But neurosis, insofar as the repressed has been victorious in it, must bring back the primeval picture.

[1.] Our first hypothesis would thus maintain that mankind, under the influence of the privations that the encroaching Ice Age imposed upon it,

22. Fritz Wittels (1912); see esp. pp. 1–19.

23. In the manuscript (p. 11, l. 22) Ferenczi's name is underlined. In fair copies intended for publication, Freud habitually distinguished names for the printer by underscoring them.

24. ⟨Here, as elsewhere, Freud uses the plural *Eiszeiten* (Ice Ages) instead of the more usual singular form.⟩

25. In the manuscript (p. 11, l. 38), a crossed-out *sehen* (see) precedes *erkennen* (recognize).

has become generally *anxious*. The hitherto predominantly friendly outside world, which bestowed every satisfaction, transformed itself into a mass of threatening perils. There had been good reason for realistic anxiety about everything new. The sexual libido, to be sure, did not at first lose its objects, which are certainly human; but it is conceivable that the ego, whose existence was threatened, to some extent abandoned the object-cathexis,[26] retained the libido in the ego, and thus transformed into realistic anxiety what had previously been object-libido. Now we see in infantile anxiety that, when satisfaction is denied, the child transforms the object-libido into realistic anxiety about strangers, but we also see that it is generally inclined to be fearful of anything new. We have carried on a long dispute over whether realistic anxiety or anxiety of longing[27] is the earlier of the two; whether the child changes his libido into realistic anxiety because he regards [it] as too great, dangerous, and thus arrives at an idea of danger, or whether he rather yields to a general anxiousness and learns from this also to be afraid of his unsatisfied libido. We were inclined to assume the former, to give precedence to longing anxiety, but we were lacking a particular disposition. We had to explain it as a generally child-like inclination. Now phylogenetic consideration seems to settle this dispute in favor of realistic anxiety and permits us to assume that a portion of the children bring along the anxiousness of the beginning of the Ice Age and are now induced by it to treat the unsatisfied libido as an external danger. The relative excess of libido would result from the same set of conditions, however, and make possible new acquisition of the disposed anxiousness. Still, the discussion of anxiety hysteria would support the preponderance of the phylogenetic disposition over all other factors.

2. As the hard times progressed, the primal humans, whose existence was threatened, must have been subjected to the conflict between self-preservation and desire to procreate, which finds its expression in most of the typical[28] cases of hysteria. Food was not sufficient to permit an increase in the human hordes, and the powers of the individual were not adequate to keep so many helpless beings alive. The killing of newborn infants

26. At this point in the manuscript (p. 13, l. 1) there is no comma, but rather a crossed-out *und* (and).

27. ⟨This term *Sehnsuchtangst* appears only once in Freud's published work, in *The Ego and the Id* (1923b, p. 58).⟩

28. This word *typischen* is written in the manuscript (p. 14, l. 7) after *Fällen* (cases) but is then transposed to the correct place.

certainly found a resistance in the love especially of the narcissistic[29] mothers. Accordingly, it became a social obligation to limit reproduction. Perverse satisfactions that did not lead to the propagation of children avoided this prohibition, which promoted a certain regression to the phase of the libido before the primacy of the genitals. The limitation must have affected[30] women more severely than men, who were less concerned about the consequences of sexual intercourse. This whole situation obviously corresponds to the conditions of conversion hysteria. From its symptomatology we conclude that man was still speechless when, because of an emergency beyond his control, he imposed the prohibition of reproduction on himself, thus also had not yet built up the system of the Pcs. over his Ucs. Those who are disposed to conversion hysteria then also regress to it, especially women, under the influence of prohibitions that want to eliminate the genital function, while intensely exciting early impressions press for genital activity.

3. The subsequent evolution is easy to construct. It primarily affected the male. After he had learned to economize on his libido and by means of regression to degrade his sexual activity to an earlier phase, activating his intelligence became paramount for him. He learned how to investigate, how to understand the hostile world[31] somewhat, and how by means of inventions to secure his first mastery over it. He developed himself under the sign of energy, formed the beginnings of language, and had to assign great significance to the new acquisitions. Language was magic to him, his thoughts seemed omnipotent to him, he understood the world according to his ego. It is the time of the animistic world view and its magical trappings. As a reward for his power to safeguard the lives of so many other helpless ones he bestowed upon himself unrestrained dominance over them, and through his personality established the first two tenets that he was himself invulnerable and that his possession of women must not be challenged. At the end of this epoch the human race had disintegrated into

29. In the same way as described in the previous note *narzißtischen* (narcissistic) is here inserted in the manuscript (p. 14, l. 15).

30. At this point in the manuscript (p. 14), the word *Abstinenz* (abstinence) is visible between ll. 22 and 23.

31. Here in the original (p. 15, ll. 11–12) is written *Welt feindliche* (world hostile); that is, as he was writing, Freud again inserted the adjective after the noun, but this time failed to transpose the two words.

individual hordes that were dominated by a strong and wise[32] brutal man as father. It is possible that the egoistically jealous and inconsiderate nature that we from ethnopsychological considerations attribute to the primal father of the human horde was not present from the beginning, but rather was developed in the course of the severe Ice Age as a result of adaptation to exigency.

Now obsessional neurosis recapitulates the characteristics of this phase of mankind, some in a negative way, because neurosis does after all [in the form of its] reaction formations,[33] correspond to the struggle against this return. The overemphasis on thinking, the enormous energy that returns in[34] the compulsion, the omnipotence of thoughts, the inclination to inviolable laws[35] are unchanged features. But against the brutal impulses that want to replace love life, there arises the resistance of later developments, which from the libidinal conflict finally saps the life energy of the individual and leaves standing, leaves [over] as compulsion, only the impulses that have been displaced to trivialities. So this human type, so valuable for the development of civilization, perishes in its return from the demands of love life, just as the grandiose type of the primal father himself, who later returned as godhead, has perished in reality from the familial relationships he created for himself.

4. We might have come so far in completing a program envisioned by Ferenczi "to bring the neurotic types of regression into harmony with the stages of human phylogeny,"[36] perhaps without straying into all-too-risky speculations. We would have no clue to the subsequent and later-appearing narcissistic neuroses, however, if the assumption did not come to our aid that the disposition to them had been acquired by a second generation, whose development introduces a new phase of human civilization.

32. In the manuscript (p. 15, l. 33) Freud added *weisen* (wise) in the margin and marked that this word should come before *brutalen* (brutal).

33. On p. 16, l. 9 *Reaktionsbildgen* (reaction formations), at the beginning of the line, is placed diagonally over *diese Wiederkehr* (this return). Freud did not indicate where the word should be inserted.

34. Freud first wrote *als* (as) (p. 16, l. 11), which he later crossed out and replaced with *im* (in).

35. The fourth element of the series, *die Neigung zu unverbrüchlichen Gesetzen* (the inclination to inviolable laws), occurred to Freud somewhat later. As was his custom, he inserted it in the continuing text—here attached to *Entwicklungen* (developments)—circled it, and moved it to the correct location. See the facsimile, p. 16, ll. 12–17.

36. Ferenczi (1913, p. 236). The actual quotation reads somewhat differently: "It is to be assumed that we shall some day succeed in bringing the individual stages in the development of the ego, and the neurotic regression-types of these, into a parallel."

This second generation begins with the sons, to whom the jealous primal father does not allow full scope. We have indicated elsewhere (*T and T*)[37] that he drives them out when they reach the age of puberty. ΨA experiences admonish us, however, to substitute another, more gruesome solution—namely, that he robs them of their manhood—after which they are able to stay in the horde as harmless laborers. We may imagine the effect of castration in that primeval time as an extinguishing of the libido and a standstill in individual development. Such a state seems to be recapitulated by dementia praecox, which especially as hebephrenia leads to giving up every love-object, degeneration of all sublimations, and return to auto-erotism. The youthful individual behaves as though he had undergone castration. In fact, self-castrations are not uncommon with this disorder. One should not bring into the phylogenetic picture what otherwise characterizes this illness, the speech alterations and hallucinatory storms, because they represent restitutive attempts, the numerous efforts to regain the object, which in the clinical picture are [for a] while[38] almost more noticeable than the phenomena of degeneration.

The assumption that the sons were treated in this way is related to a question that should be answered in passing. Where does replacement of and succession to the primal fathers come from when they get rid of the sons in such a way?[39] Atkinson [1903] already showed the way when he pointed out that only the older sons had to fear the full persecution of the father, but the youngest—schematically considered—thanks to the intercession of the mother, but mainly as a consequence of the father's aging and his need to be helped, had the prospect of eluding this fate and becoming the father's successor. This advantage of the youngest was totally eliminated in the subsequent social configuration and was replaced by the prerogative of the oldest. In myth and fairy tale, however, it remains highly recognizable.

5. The next change could only consist in the fact that the threatened sons avoided castration by means of flight and, allied with one another, learned to take upon themselves the struggle for survival. This living

37. *Totem and Taboo* (1912–13).

38. The word *Zeitlang* is added in the margin of the original (p. 17, l. 37). From the way it is written it is not clear where Freud wanted to put it.

39. In connection with this see Freud's indication in the accompanying letter (above) that Ferenczi's objection has been taken into consideration. For further details consult the essay "Metapsychology and Metabiology" later in this volume.

together had to bring social feelings to the fore and could have been built upon homosexual sexual satisfaction. It is very possible that the long-sought hereditary disposition of homosexuality can be glimpsed in the inheritance of this phase of the human condition.[40] The social feelings that originated here, sublimated from homosexuality, became mankind's lasting possession, however, and the basis for every later society. This phase of the condition, however, manifestly brings back paranoia; more correctly, paranoia defends itself against its return. In ⟨paranoia⟩ secret alliances are not lacking, and the persecutor plays a tremendous role. Paranoia tries to ward off homosexuality, which was the basis for the organization of brothers, and in so doing must drive the victim out of society and[41] destroy his social sublimations.

6. Ranking melancholia-mania in this context seems to encounter the difficulty that a normal time for the individual appearance of this neurotic[42] illness cannot be determined with certainty. But it is definite that it belongs to the age of maturity rather than to that of childhood. If one looks at the characteristic alternation of depression and elation, it is difficult not to recall the very similar succession of triumph and mourning that forms a regular component of religious festivities: mourning over the death of the god, triumphal joy over his resurrection. This religious ceremony, however, as we have surmised from the statements of ethnopsychology, only recapitulates in reverse the attitude of the members of the brother clan after they have overpowered[43] and killed the primal father: triumph over his death, then mourning over the fact that they all still revered him as a model. So might this great event of human history, which made an end of the primal horde and replaced it with the victorious organization of brothers, provide the predisposition for the peculiar succession of moods that we acknowledge as a particular narcissistic disorder alongside the paraphrenias. The mourning about[44] the primal father pro-

40. ⟨The German word is *Zustandsphase*. In his letter to Ferenczi of July 12, 1915, translated by Ernest Jones (p. 79), Freud writes *Zustandsphasen der Menschheit,* which Jones translates as "phases in human conditions."⟩

41. In the manuscript (p. 19, l. 10) this *und* (and) is located at the end of the paragraph. Presumably Freud wanted to enter it at the above location, but there is no arrow.

42. "Neurotic" in this instance is used, obviously, in the sense of psychoneurosis, not of transference neurosis.

43. Here (p. 19, l. 32) Freud first wrote *überfallen* (attacked), then crossed out *fallen* and wrote *wältigt* ⟨that is, *überwaltigt* (overpowered)⟩.

44. Freud first wrote *über* (over), then *um* (about) (p. 20, l. 6).

ceeds from identification with him, and such identification we have established[45] as the prerequisite for the melancholic mechanism.

To summarize, we can say: If the dispositions to the three transference neuroses were acquired in the struggle with the exigencies of the Ice Age, then the fixations that underlie the narcissistic neuroses originate from the oppression by the father, who after the end of the Ice Age assumes, continues its role, as it were,[46] against the second generation. As the first struggle leads to the patriarchal stage of civilization, the second ⟨leads⟩ to the social; but from both come the fixations which in their return after millennia become the disposition of the two groups of neuroses. Also in this sense neurosis is therefore a cultural acquisition. The parallel that has been sketched here may be no more than a playful comparison. The extent to which it may throw light on the still unsolved riddles of the neuroses should properly be left to further investigation, and illumination through new experiences.[47]

Now it is time to think [about a] series of objections, which caution us not to overestimate the reconstructions we have arrived at. First, it [will become] obvious to everyone that the second series of dispositions, those of the second generation, can only be acquired by men (as sons), whereas dementia praecox, paranoia, and melancholia can just as well be produced by women. Women in primal times lived under even more diverse conditions than they do today. Furthermore, there is attached to these dispositions a difficulty of which those [of the] first series are free: they appear to be acquired under conditions that exclude heredity. It is evident that the castrated and intimidated sons do not procreate, therefore cannot pass on their disposition (dementia praecox). Similarly, the ψ condition of the banished sons, bound together in homosexuality, cannot influence the next generations, for they die out as infertile branches of the family, as long as they have not triumphed over the father. But if they do achieve

45. This was in "Mourning and Melancholia" (1917e [1915]), one of the other metapsychological papers of 1915, which had already been completed when Freud was composing the present draft.

46. This *gleichsam* (as it were), evidently jotted down later, is located in the left margin of the manuscript (p. 20, l. 19). There is no clear indication of where Freud wanted to insert it.

47. At this point (p. 20, l. 35) is a fairly long horizontal line, Freud's sign for the end of the manuscript. What follows is the addition announced in the accompanying letter (pp. xvi-xvii above), a reaction to Ferenczi's letter. For additional details see pp. 80–81.

this triumph, then it is one generation's experience that must be denied the necessary unlimited reproduction.

As one can imagine, we need not be at a loss for particulars in such obscure areas. The difficulty basically coincides with one that has been posed earlier, namely, how the brutal father of the Ice Age, who was certainly not immortal like his divine image, reproduced himself. Again there appears the younger son, who later becomes a father—who, to be sure, is not castrated himself, but knows the fate of his older brothers and fears it for himself; he must have been tempted, like the more fortunate of them, to flee and to renounce women. So next to those men who fall by the wayside as infertile, there may remain a chain of others, who in their person go through the vicissitudes of the male sex and can propagate them as dispositions. The essential point of view remains firm, that for him [the younger son] the oppression of the father replaces the exigencies of the time.

The triumph over the father must have been planned and fantasized through countless generations before it was realized. How the dispositions produced by the father's oppression spread to women seems in itself to create greater difficulties. The vicissitudes of women in these primeval times are especially obscure to us. Thus, conditions of life that we have not recognized may come into consideration. But we are spared the grossest difficulty by observing that we should not forget human bisexuality. Thus women can assume the dispositions acquired by men and bring them to light in themselves.

In the meantime let us make it clear that with these particulars we have basically done no more than save our scientific fantasies from being criticized as absurd. On the whole, they retain their value as a salutary rude awakening if we were perhaps on [the] way to placing the phylogenetic disposition above everything else. Thus, it does not[48] come about that archaic constitutions return in new individuals according to a predetermined ratio and force them into neurosis through conflict with the demands of the present. There remains room for new acquisition and for influences with which we are not acquainted. In sum, we are not at the end, but rather at the beginning, of an understanding of this phylogenetic factor.

48. This *nicht* (not) was perhaps subsequently placed at the beginning of p. 22, l. 37.

Übersicht der Übertragungsneurosen

SIGMUND FREUD

Facsimile and Transcription

Note on the Facsimile

The manuscript was folded in half inside the envelope (also shown in facsimile), which was addressed to Sándor Ferenczi, marked "Registered," and carried the appropriate postal sticker. The corner bearing the postage stamp was torn off and is missing; along with it, several letters of an address were removed. From the remnants that are recognizable in the facsimile, one might conclude that Freud originally had planned to give the script to someone who intended to visit Ferenczi. (At first glance, "Miss Do——" suggests the American writer Hilda Doolittle, with whom, however, Freud was not yet acquainted.) The meaning of the other scribblings on the envelope is unclear.

The manuscript, written in ink on both sides of the page, measures 21.3 by 33.7 centimeters. (Its size in the facsimile is therefore reduced.) Freud noted each page number with a reddish-brown colored pencil. The diagonal lines with which the individual blocks of text are crossed out also are reddish-brown in the original. Freud presumably marked the passages in this way as soon as he had successively taken them into account in the fair copy—which, as he emphasizes in the accompanying letter to Ferenczi (on the reverse of the last page of the manuscript and also reproduced in facsimile), followed the draft "sentence for sentence." The words, letters, and abbreviations set sans serif in the transcription are written in the manuscript in Latin letters.

I.G.-S.

XII Übersicht der Übertraggsneurosen

Vorbereitung.

Nach Detailuntersuchg versuchen Charaktere zusam̄enfassen, Abgrenzg von anderen, vergleichende Durchführg der einzelnen Momente. Momente sind: Verdrgg, Ersatz u Symptbildung, (Gegenbesetzung), Verhältnis z. Sexualfunktion Regression, Disposition. Beschränken auf die 3 Typen Angsthy, Konvhy und Zw.

a) Vdgg. findet bei allen 3 an Grenze des ubw u vbw Systems statt, besteht in Abziehung oder Verweigerung vbw Besetzung, wird gesichert durch Art von Gegenbesetzung. Bei Zw in späteren Stadien verschiebt sie sich auf Grenze zwischen Vbw u Bw.

Werden hören, daß in nächster Gruppe die Vdgg, andere Topik hat, sie erweitert sich dann zum Begriff d. Spaltung.

Topische Gesichtspunkt darf nicht in dem Sinn überschätzt werden, daß etwa jeder Verkehr zwischen beiden Systemen durch sie unterbrochen würde. Es wird also wesentlicher an welchen Elementen diese Schranke eingeführt wird.

Erfolg u Abgeschloßenheit

hängen insof zusam̄en, als Miserfolg zu weiteren Bemühungen nötigt. Erfolg variirt bei den 3 Neurosen u in einzel Stadien derselben.

Erfolg am geringsten bei Angsthy, beschränkt sich darauf, daß keine vbw u (bw) Repraesentanz zu Stande kom̄t. Später, daß anstatt der anstößigen eine Ersatz vbw u bw wird. Endlich bei Phobiebildg erreicht er Zweck, in Hem̄g des Unlustaffekts

XII. Übersicht der Übertragungsneurosen

Vorbereitung.

Die Unterscheidung der einzelnen Momente auseinanderzuhalten, Übergang von einander, vergleichende Dignität der einzelnen Momente.

Momente sind: Verdrängung, Ersatz- u Symptombildung, Gegenbesetzung, Fixierung, Konversion, Regression, Disposition. Beschränken uns auf die 3 Typen Angsthy., Konvhy. und Zw.N.

a) Vdg. findet bei allen dreien an der Grenze des Ubw Systems statt, besteht in Abziehung der vorbewußten Besetzung, wird gesichert durch [illegible] Gegenbesetzung. Sie [illegible] in späteren Stadien vielleicht an der Grenze zwischen Vbw u Bw.

Werden später [illegible] in nächster Stunde die [illegible] andere Logik [illegible] nicht [illegible] zum Begriff d. Spaltung.

Logischer Gesichtspunkt darf nicht in dem Sinne überschätzt werden, daß einer oder der andere zwischen beiden Systemen durch [illegible] werden. [illegible] an welchen Stellen [illegible] eingesetzt wird.

Erfolg u Zweckmäßigkeit.

[illegible] nicht [illegible] als Mißerfolg zu [illegible] Erfolg [illegible] bei den 3 Neurosen u im späteren Stadium derselben.

Erfolg am geringsten bei Angsthy., beschränkt sich darauf, daß keine Vbw [illegible] Besetzung [illegible] Stand hält, dafür der [illegible] einen Ersatz aber [illegible] Bw wird, endlich bei Phobiebildung [illegible], [illegible] der Unlustaffekts

2 durch großen Verzicht, ausgiebig Fluchtversuch.

~~Z~~ Absicht der Vdgg ist im̄er Unlustvermeidg.

Schicksal der Repraesentanz ist nur ein Zeichen des Vorgangs. Die scheinbare (deskriptiv, statt syst.) Zerlegg des abzuwehrenden Vorgangs in Vorstellg und Affekt (Repraes. u quantit Faktor) ergiebt sich eben daraus, daß Vdgg in Verweigerg der Wortvorstellg besteht, also aus topisch Charakter der Vdgg.

Bei Zw ist Erfolg zuerst ein voller, aber kein dauernder. Prozeß noch weniger abgeschloßen Er setzt sich nach erster erfolgreicher Phase durch zwei weitere fort, von denen erstere (sek. Vdgg) sich wie Angsthy mit Ersetzg der Repraesentanz begnügt, spätere (tertiäre) der Phobie entsprech. Verzichte u Einschränkg produzirt aber zum Unterschied mit logisch Mitteln arbeitet.

Im Gegensatz hiezu ist Erfolg der Konversshy von Anfang ein ein voller, aber durch starke Ersatzbildg erkaufter. Prozeß des einzeln Vdggvorgangs abgeschloßener.

Bildg der Zwvorstellg. Kampf geg. Zwvorstellg

b) ~~Ersatz u Symptombildg~~ Gegenbesetzung

Bei Angsthy fehlt sie zuerst reiner Fluchtversuch, wirft sich dan̄ auf Ersatzvorstellg u bes. in dritter Phase auf Umgebg derselben, um von da aus Bändigg der Unlustentbindg zu sichern, als Wachsamkeit Aufmerksamkeit. Repraesentirt den Anteil der vbw, also den Aufwand, den Neurose kostet.

Bei Zw, wo es sich von Anfang um Abwehr eines ambivalent Trieb handelt, besorgt sie die erste glückende Vdgg, leistet dann Reaktionsbildung dank der Ambivalenz giebt dann in tertiärer Phase die Aufmerk

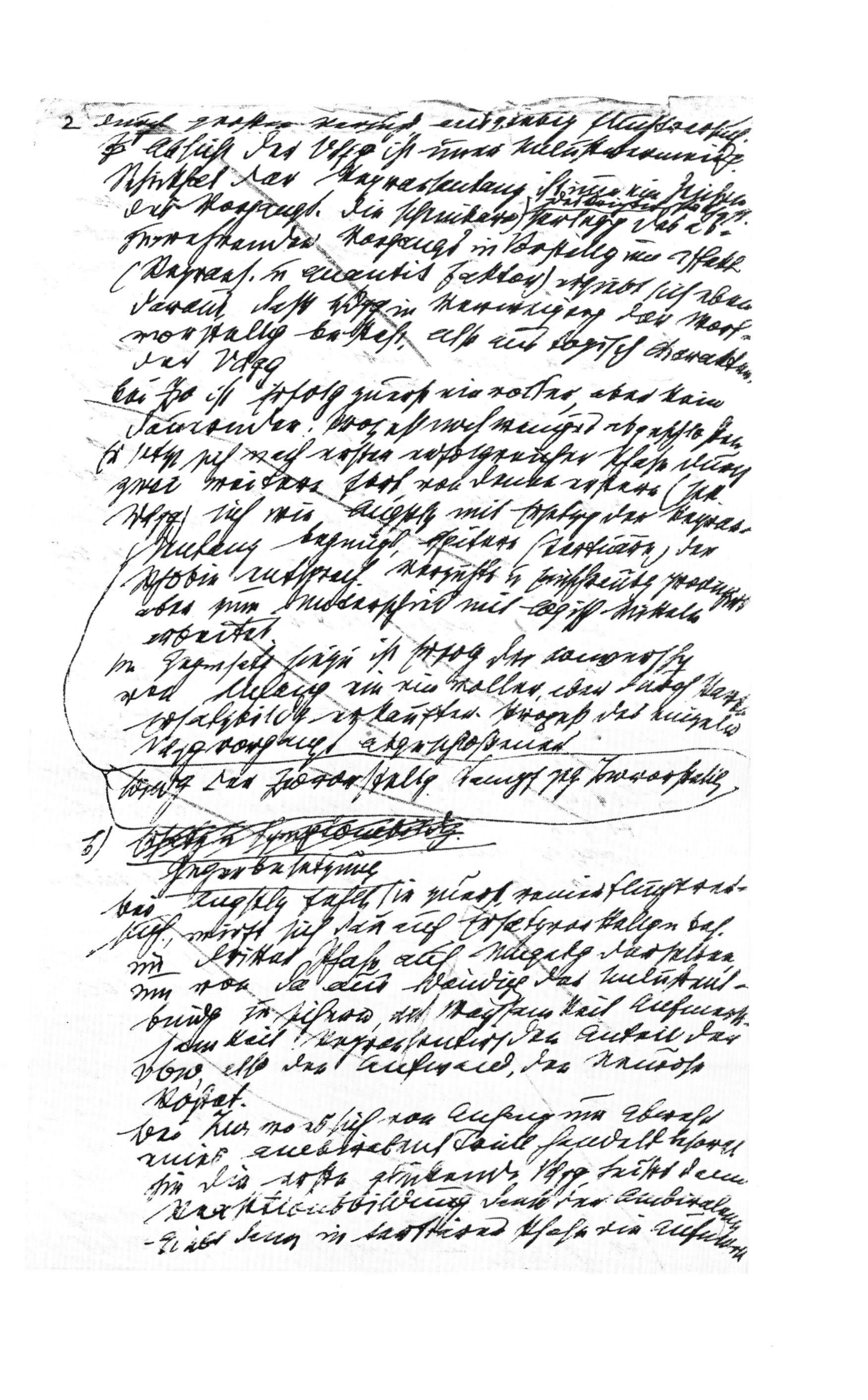

2 [illegible]

[illegible]

b) [illegible]

[illegible]

3 samkeit, die Zwvorst. auszeichnet u besorgt die logische Arbeit, also 2 u 3 Phase ganz wie bei Angst Unterschied in 1 Phase, wo bei Angst nichts, bei Zw alles leistet.

Im̄er sichert sie Vdgg entsp Anteil des Vbw.

Bei Hy glückl Charakter dadurch ermöglicht, daß Gegenbes von Anfang an Zusam̄entreffen mit Triebbesetzg sucht u sich zum Kompromiß mit ihr einigt, auswälende Bestim̄g auf Repraesentanz trifft.

c) Ersatz u Symptombildg.

Entspricht der Wiederkehr Vdgten, Mislingen der Vdgg. Eine Weile zu sondern, später fließt mit ihr zusam̄en.

am vollkom̄ensten bei Konvhy: Ersatz = Symptom, nichts weiter zu trennen.

Ebenso bei Angsthy, Ersatzbildg ermöglicht dem Vdgt die erste Wiederkehr.

Bei Zw sondert sich scharf, indem erste Ersatzbildg von Verdrgend durch Gegenbesetzg geliefert u nicht zu Symptomen gerechnet wird. Dafür sind späteren Symptome der Zw. oft vorwiegend Wiederkehr des verdrängten, Anteil des Verdrgd an ihnen geringer.

Symtombildg, von der unser Studium ausgeht, fällt im̄er mit Wiederkehr des Vdgten zusam̄en u geschieht mit Hilfe der Regression und der disponirenden Fixirungen.

Ein allgem. Gesetz sagt aus, daß die Regression bis zur Fixirg zurückgeht und von dort aus Wiederkehr des Verdrängten sich durchsetzt

d) Verhältnis z. Sexualfunktion

Für dies bleibt bestehen, daß verdrgte Triebregung stets eine libidinöse dem Sexualleben angehörige ist.

3 [illegible]arbeit, die bewusst [illegible] u. bewusste
logische Arbeit. Also 2te Phase ganz wie das
[illegible] unterschied in [illegible], wo bei Angsth.
mehr das Ich alles leistet.
[illegible] zu Weg [illegible] das [illegible]
bei Hy [illegible] Bedeutung [illegible]
daß Gegenbes. von Anfang an [illegible]
mit [illegible] u. [illegible] Kompromiß
mit ihr [illegible] [illegible] Bedeutung auf
[illegible].

c) Ersatz u. Symptombildung.

Entspricht der Wiederkehr des Verdrängten, Mißlingen
der Vdg. [illegible] später [illegible]
mit ihr zusammen.
Angstersatz bei Angsthy: Ersatz-
symptom nicht weiter zu trennen
[illegible] Ersatzbildung vermutlich
[illegible] Wiederkehr.
[illegible] ändert sich später, indem erste Ersatzbildung von [illegible] Gegenbesetzung [illegible] u. nicht zu Symptomen gerechnet
wird. [illegible] späteren Symptome der Wiederkehr [illegible] Anteil des Verdrängten an ihrer Gestaltung.
[illegible]
Symptombildung [illegible] Wiederkehr des [illegible]
[illegible] mit [illegible]
[illegible] u. [illegible]
[illegible]
[illegible]
[illegible]
[illegible]

d) Verhältnis z. Sexualfunktion

[illegible]
[illegible]
[illegible]

4 während Verdrgg vom Ich ausgeht aus verschiedenen Motiven, die sich als ein nicht Können (wegen Uberstärke) oder Nichtwollen zusam̄enfassen laßen. Das letztere geht auf Unverträglichkeit mit den Ichidealen oder auf andersartige befürchtete Schädigg des Ichs zurück. Das Nichtkönnen entspricht auch einer Schädigg.

Verdunkelt wird diese fundamentale Thatsache durch zwei Momente, erstens hat es oft Anschein, als ob Vdgg durch Konflikt zweier Regungen beide libidinös sind angeregt würde. Dies löst sich durch die Erwagg, daß die eine davon ichgerecht ist u in dem Konflikt die Hilfe der vom Ich ausgehenden Vdgg anrufen kann. Zweitens, indem nicht nur libid sondern auch Ichstrebg unter den verdrängt angetroffen werden, bes. haufig u deutlich bei längerem Bestand und fortgeschritt Entwicklg der Neurose. Letztere kom̄t so zu Stande, daß die vdgte lib. Regung sich auf dem Umweg durch eine Ichstrebg, der sie eine Komponente geliehen hat, durchzusetzen sucht, ihr Energie überträgt und nun diese mit in die Vdgg reißt, was im großen Umfange geschehen kann. An Allgemeingiltigkeit jenes Satzes wird dadurch nichts geändert. Begreifliche Forderg. daß man Einsichten aus den Anfangsstadien der Neurosen schöpfe, Bei Hy und Zw evident, daß sich Vdgg gegen ~~das~~ die Sexualfunktion in definitiver Form, in der es Anspruch der Fortpflanzung repraesentirt richtet. Am deutlichsten wieder bei Konversionshy weil ohne Komplikationen, bei Zw erst Regression. Indeß diese Beziehg nicht über-

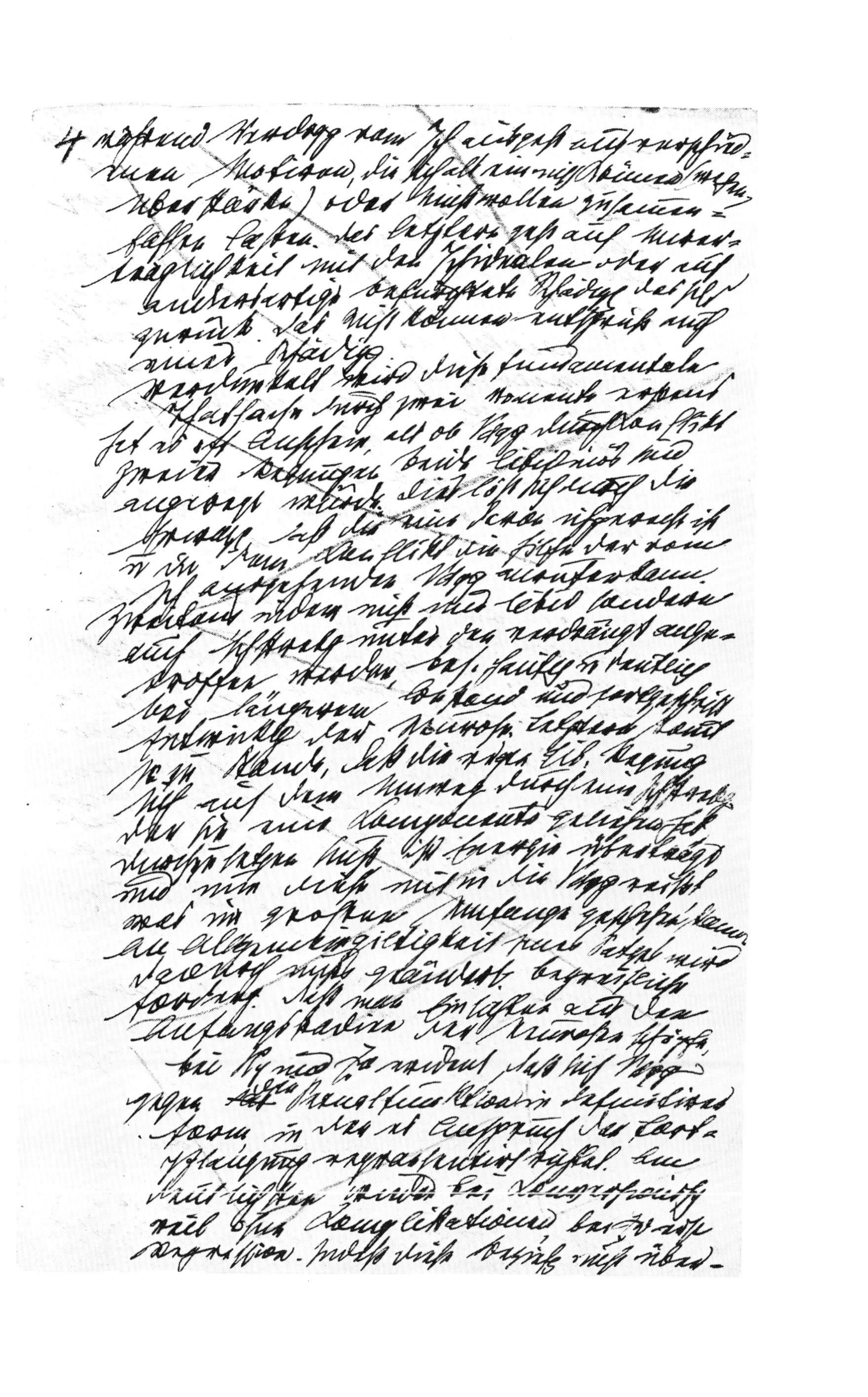

4

5 treiben, nicht etwa annehmen, daß Vdgg erst mit diesem Stadium der Libido in Wirksamkeit tritt. Im Gegenteil zeigt ja gerade Zw, daß Vdgg allgemeiner Vorgang, nicht libidinös abhängig weil hier gegen Vorstufe gerichtet. Ebenso in Entwicklg, daß Vdgg auch gegen perverse Reggen in Anspruch genom̄en. Frage, warum Vdgg hier gelingt, sonst nicht, in Natur libid Strebg sehr vertretgsfähig, so daß bei Vdgg der normal die perversen verstärkt werden u umgekehrt. Zur Sexualfunkt. Vdgg kein anderes Verhältnis, als daß sie zu ihrer Abwehr bemüht wird wie Regression u andere Triebschicksale.

Bei Angsthy ist Verhaltnis zur Sexualf. undeutlicher aus Gründ, die bei Behandlg der Angst zum Vorschein gekom̄en. Scheint, daß Angsthy jene Falle umfaßt, in denen Sextriebanspruch als zu groß wie Gefahr abgewehrt. Keine bes. Bedingg aus Libidoorganisation.

e) Regression. Das interessanteste Moment und Triebschicksal. Von Angsthy aus keinen Anlaß es zu erraten. Könnte sagen, daß hier nicht in Betracht kom̄t, vielleicht weil jede spätere Angsthy so deutlich auf eine infantile regredirt (die vorbildliche Disposition der N) und diese letztere so frühzeitig im Leben auftritt. Dagegen die beiden anderen schönste Beispiele von Regression, aber diese spielt bei jeder andere Rolle in Struktur der Neurose. Bei Convhy ist es eine starke Ichregression, Rückkehr zu Phase ohne Scheidg von Vbw und Ubw, also ohne Sprache und Zensur. Die Regression dient aber der Symptombildg u Wiederkehr des Vdgt. Die Triebregung die vom

5 werden nicht etwa annehmen, daß Vdg erst mit
welchem Stadium der Libido in Wirksamkeit
tritt. Im Gegenteil zeigt sie gerade so, daß Vdg
allgemeiner Vorgang mit Libido an anfänglich
weil sie gegen Objekte gerichtet. Hierdurch
entwickelt daß Vdg auch gegen spätere Regungen
in Anspruch genommen. Frage, warum Vdg
hier gelingt kommt nicht in Libido-Leben
Vorbeugen sehr unverständlich, so daß bei
Vdg der Wandel des Charakters ersparte
werden, in eingeleitet und Libidoschicksal
Vdg kann anderes Verfallens, als daß die
zu [illegible] abzulenken [illegible] wird die Regression
an andern Teile [illegible]
bei Angsthy ist Verhältnis der Libidobedürftigkeit
auf Grund der bei besonders der Angst einer
Vorbereitung gekommen. Hinweis, daß Angsthy jenes
Falles umfaßt in deren Lebensäußerung
als zu groß und sehr allgemein [illegible]
[illegible] auf Libidoregungen [illegible]

e) Regression. Ist das interessanteste Moment und
Triebschicksal. Der Angsthy läßt keinen Anlaß
zu verraten. Darunter sagen, daß sie nicht im
Verlauf [illegible] weil jede spätere
Angsthy so deutlich auf einen infantilen Vorgang
(die ursprüngliche Disposition der Angst [illegible]
nicht [illegible] so frühzeitig im Leben auftritt.
Dagegen die beiden anderen Neurosen Beispiele von Regression aber diese spielt
bei jeder [illegible] Rolle im Zustand
der Neurose. Bei Konvhy ist es eine starke
Regression, Rückkehr zu [illegible] ohne
[illegible] von Obw und Ubw also ohne
Sprache und Zensur. Die Regression [illegible]
[illegible] der Symptombildung [illegible]
des [illegible] die [illegible]

6 aktuellen Ich nicht akzeptirt, rekurrirt auf ein früheres, von dem aus sie Abfuhr freilich in anderer Weise findet. Daß es dabei virtuell zu einer Art Libidoregress kom̄t, schon erwähnt. Bei Zw ist es anders. Die Regression ist eine Libidoregression, dient nicht der Wiederkehr sondern der Vdgg u wird durch eine starke konstit Fixirg oder unvollkom̄ene Ausbildg ermöglicht. In der That fällt hier erster Schritt der Abwehr der Regression zu, wo es sich mehr um Regression als auf Entwicklgshem̄g handelt, und die regressive libidin Organis unterliegt dann erst einer typischen Verdrängg, die aber erfolglos bleibt. Ein Stück Ichregression wird von der Libido aus Ich aufgezwungen oder ist in der unvollkom̄enen Entwicklg des Ichs, die hier mit Libphase zusam̄enhängt, gegeben. (Tren̄g d. Ambivalenzen) f). Hinter Regression verhüllen sich die Probleme der Fixirung u Disposition. Die Regression kann man allgemein sagen reicht so weit zurück bis zu einer Fixirungsstelle, entweder in Ich- oder Libentwicklg., u diese stellt die Disposition dar. Dies ist also das maßgebendste, die Entscheidg über Neurosenwal vermittelnde Moment. Lohnt also dabei zu verweilen. Fixirung kom̄t durch Phase d. Entwicklg zu Stande, die zu stark ausgeprägt war oder vielleicht auch zu lange angehalten hat, um restlos in die nächste überzugehen. Klarere Vorstellg, worin, in welchen

6 [illegible] nicht abgestreift, vielmehr
auf ein [illegible]
freilich in anderer Weise findet. [illegible]
dabei [illegible]
[illegible] Man erwartet [illegible]
anders. Die Regression ist eine Libidoregression, [illegible]
[illegible]
[illegible]
[illegible]
[illegible]
Regression [illegible]
[illegible]
[illegible]
[illegible]
[illegible]
[illegible]
[illegible]
[illegible]
[illegible]
[illegible]
Problems: die Fixierung u. Disposition
die Regression. Denn man allgemein
sagen kann, je weiter [illegible] einer
Fixierungsstelle [illegible]
überentwickelt, [illegible] Stelle die Disposition
der. [illegible]
[illegible]
[illegible] Moment. [illegible]
Fixierung [illegible] Entwicklg
[illegible]
[illegible]
[illegible]
[illegible]

7 Veränderg die Fixirg besteht, wird am besten nicht verlangen. Aber über Herkunft etwas sagen. Besteht sowol die Möglichkeit, daß solche Fixirg rein mitgebracht sowie daß sie durch frühzeitige Eindrücke herbeigeführt und endlich, daß beide Faktoren zusam̄enwirken. Umsomehr da man behaupten darf, beiderlei Momente seien eigentlich ubiquitär, da alle Dispositionen konstitutionell vorhanden sind im Kinde u anderseits die wirksamen Eindrücke sehr vielen Kindern gleicher Weise zu teil werden. Handelt sich also um mehr oder weniger und ein wirksames Zusam̄entreffen. Da niemand konstit. Momente bestreiten geneigt ist, fällt es ΨA zu auch das Anrecht der frühinfantil Erwerbg kraftig zu vertreten. Bei Zw ist übrigens das konstit Moment weit deutlicher erkannt, als bei KHy das akzidentelle, das ist zuzugeben. Detailverteilg im̄er noch zweifelhaft.

Wo das konstit Moment der Fixirung in Betracht kom̄t, damit Erwerbg nicht beseitigt, sie rückt nur in noch frühere Vorzeit, da man mit Recht behaupten darf, daß die ererbten Dispositionen Reste der Erwerbung der Vorahnen sind. Hiemit stößt man an Problem der phylogenetischen Disposition hinter der individuell oder ontogenetischen, und darf keinen Widerspruch finden, wenn das Individ zu seiner ererbten Disposition auf Grund früheren Erlebens neue Dispositionen aus eigenem Erleben hinzufügt. Warum sollte der

7 Veränderung die häufig besteht, wiederum besser nicht verlangen. Man aber fast nicht [illegible] sehen. Besteht immer die Möglichkeit, daß solche Steigerung mitgebracht, sowie daß sie auch farbige Eindrücke hervorge- führt und endlich, daß beide Faktoren zusammenwirken. Insofern da man an- fangen darf, beiderlei Momente seien eigentlich überflüssig, da alle Dispositionen konstitutionelle vorhanden sind um durch anderseits den wirksamen Eindrücke [illegible] vielen Hörern glaubhaft zu Teil werden. Handelt sich also um mehr oder weniger und um wirksames Zusammen- treffen. Da niemand konstit. Momente [illegible] geneigt ist, fällt es ihm auch das Moment der [illegible] Erwartung [illegible] zu verlassen. [illegible] ist [illegible] das konstit. Moment [illegible] [illegible] als [illegible] ist [illegible] noch zweifelhaft. Als das konstit. Moment das [illegible] [illegible] dadurch [illegible] nicht bestätigt, [illegible] noch [illegible] vorzüglich [illegible] man nicht [illegible] darf, daß die [illegible] Dispositions [illegible] der Erwerbung des [illegible] sind. Damit stößt man an Probleme der phylogenetischen Disposition [illegible] individuell oder ontogenetischen, und doch keine Widerspruch [illegible] wenn das Individuum seine erworbenen Dis- position auf Grund früheren [illegible] neue Dispositionen als eigene [illegible] [illegible]. Warum sollte der

8 Prozeß, der Disposition auf Grund von Erleben schafft, gerade an dem Individ, dessen Neurose man untersucht, erlöschen? Oder dieses Disposition für seine Nachkom̄en schaffen, sie aber nicht für sich erwerben können. Scheint vielmehr notwendige Ergänzung

Wie weit die phylogenetische Disposition das Verständnis der Neuros beitragen kann, ist noch nicht zu übersehen. Es gehörte dazu auch, daß Betrachtg über enge Gebiet der Ubertraggsneuros hinausgeht. Der wichtigste unterscheidende Charakter der Ubertraggsn konnte in dieser Ubersicht ohnedieß nicht gewürdigt werden, weil er ihnen ja gemeinsam nicht auffällt und erst bei Herbeiziehg der narzißt Neuros durch Kontrast auffallen würde. ~~Er liegt in der Festhaltung des Objekts. Verhältnis des Ich zum Objekt~~. Bei dieser Vergrößerg des Horizonts würde Verhältnis von Ich zu Objekt Vordergrund rücken und Festhaltg des Objekts sich als gemeinsam Unterscheidendes ergeben. Gewiße Vorbereitung hier gestattet.

Hoffe der Leser, der sonst auch an Langweile vieler Abschnitte gemerkt hat, wie sehr alles auf sorgfältiger u mühseliger Beobachtg aufgebaut, wird Nachsicht üben, wenn auch einmal die Kritik vor der Phantasie zurücktritt u ungesicherte Dinge vorgetragen werden blos weil sie anregend sind und Blick in die Ferne eröffnen.

Es ist noch legitim anzunehmen daß auch die Neurosen Zeugnis von der seelischen Entwicklgsgeschichte des

8 Prozeß der Disposition auf Grund von früher Erlebtem geschafft gerade an dem Individ., dessen Vorfahr man unbewußt vorzufinden? Wie diese Disposition für seine Nachkommen schaffen, die aber nur bei ihm erworben können. Scheint vielmehr notwendige Ergänzung.

Wie weit die phylogenetische Disposition das Verständnis der Neurose beitragen kann, ist noch nicht zu übersehen. Es gehört dazu auch, daß Betrachtung über enge Gebiet der Übertragungsneurosen hinausgeht. Der wichtigste unterscheidende Charakter der Übertragungsneurosen konnte in dieser Übersicht eigentlich nicht gewürdigt werden, weil er ihnen gemeinsam nicht auffällt und erst bei Heranziehung der narzißtischen Neurosen durch Kontrast auffallen würde. ~~Es liegt in der Entfaltung des [illegible] narzißtischen des Ichs zum Objekt~~ Bei dieser Vergleichung der Gegensätze würde begreiflich, daß das Verhältnis von Ich zu Objekt vordergrund rücken und Schicksale des Objekts [illegible] als Neurosen unterscheidend angeben. Gewisse Vorbereitung hier gestattet.

Hoffe daß Leser, der die Langweiligkeit der Abschnitte gemerkt hat, wie sehr alles auf sorgfältigen u mühseligen Beobachtung aufgebaut wird, nachsieht wenn auch einmal die Kritik vor der Phantasie zurücktritt u unbestätigte Dinge vorgetragen werden bloß weil sie anregend sind und Blick in die Ferne eröffnen.

Es ist noch kürzlich anzumerken, daß auch die Neurosen Zeugnis von der seelischen Entwicklungsgeschichte der

9 Menschen ablegen müßen. Ich glaube nun in Aufsatz (Uber zwei Prinzipien) gezeigt zu haben, daß wir den Sexualstrebgen des Menschen eine andere Entwicklg zuschreiben dürfen als den Ichstrebgen. Der Grund wesentlich daß die ersteren ganze Weile autoerotisch befriedigt werden können, während Ichstrebgen von Anfang auf Objekt u damit auf Realität angewiesen sind. Welches die Entwicklg der menschlichen Sexuallebens glauben wir in großen Zügen gelernt zu haben (Drei Abhandlg z. Sexualtheorie) Die des menschlichen Ichs, dh der Selbsterhaltgsfunktionen u der von ihnen abgeleiteten Bildgen ist schwieriger zu durchschauen. Ich kenne nur den einzigen Versuch von Ferenczi, der ψα Erfahrungen zu diesem Zwecke verwertet. unsere Aufgabe wäre natürlich sehr erleichtert, wenn uns die Entwicklgsgeschichte des Ichs anderswoher gegeben wäre, die Neurosen zu verstehen, anstatt daß wir jetzt umgekehrt verfahren müßen. Man bekom̄t dabei den Eindruck, daß die Entwicklgsgeschichte der Libido ein weit älteres Stück der Entwicklg wiederholt als die des Ichs, erstere vielleicht Verhaltniße des Wirbeltierstam̄es wiederholt, während letztere von der Geschichte der Menschenart abhängig ist. Es existirt nun eine Reihe, an welche man verschiedene weitgehende Gedanken anknüpfen kann. Sie entsteht, wenn man die Ψneurosen (nicht die Ubertraggsneurosen allein) nach der Zeit anordnet, zu
punkt
welchem sie im individ Leben aufzutreten pflegen. Dann ist die Angsthysterie

9 Menschen ablegen mussten. Ich getraue mich im Aufsatz (Über zwei Prinzipien) gezeigt zu haben
daß wir den Sexualtrieben des Menschen
eine andere Entwicklung zuschreiben müssen
als den Ichstrebungen. Der Grundunterschied
daß die ersteren eine Weile autoerotisch
befriedigt werden können, während letztere
von Anfang an auf Objekte damit auf die
Realität angewiesen sind. Welches die
Entwicklung der menschlichen Sexualfunktion
glauben wir in großen Zügen erkannt
zu haben (drei Abhandlg. z. Sexualtheorie)
die der menschlichen Ich- oder Selbsterhaltungs-
funktionen u. der von ihnen abgeleiteten Bildungen ist schwieriger zu
durchschauen. Ich kenne nur den einzigen
Versuch von Ferenczi der ΨA Erfahrungen
zu diesem Zwecke verwertet. Unsere Aufgabe wäre natürlich sehr erleichtert
wenn uns die Entwicklungsgeschichte des
Ichs anderswoher gegeben wäre die
Neurosen zu verstehen, anstatt dass wir
jetzt umgekehrt verfahren müssen. Man
bekommt dabei den Eindruck, dass die
Entwicklungsgeschichte der Libido ein viel
älteres Stück der Entwicklung wiederholt
als die des Ichs; erstere vielleicht Ver-
hältnisse der Wirbeltierklassen
wiederholt, während letztere von der
Geschichte der Menschenart abhängig ist.
Es existiert nun eine Reihe, an welche man
weitgehende Gedanken an-
schließen kann. Sie entsteht, wenn man
die Neurosen (nicht die Übertragungsneurosen
allein) nach dem Zeitmoment, zu
welchem sie im individuellen Leben aufzutreten
pflegen. Dann ist die Angsthysterie

10 die fast voraussetzungslose die früheste, ihr schließt die Konvhy (vom 4 J etwa) an, noch etwas später in der Vorpubertät (9–10) tritt bei Kindern die Zw auf. Die narzißt. Neurosen fehlen der Kindheit. Von diesen ist die Dem pr in klassischer Form Erkrankg der Pubertätsjahre, die Par nähert sich den Jahren der Reife, und Mel-Manie auch dems. Zeitabschnitt, sonst unbestim̄bar Die Reihe lautet also:

Angsthy – Konv.hy – Zw – Dem pr – Paranoia – Die Fixirungsdispositionen – Mel-Manie dieser Affektionen scheinen auch eine Reihe zu ergeben, die aber gegenläufig ist. ~~Deutlich~~ bes. wenn man libid. Disposition in Betracht zieht. Es ergäbe sich also, je später die Neurose auftritt, auf desto frühere Libidophase muß sie regrediren. Dies gilt indeß nur in großen Zügen. Unzweifelhaft richtet sich Khy gegen Primat d. Genitalien die Zw gegen die sadist. Vorstufe, alle 3 Übertraggsneuros gegen vollzogene Libidoentwicklg. Die narzißt Neuros aber gehen auf Phasen vor Objektfindg zurück, die Dem pr regredirt bis zum Autoerotis die Paranoia bis zur narzißt homosex. Objektwal, der Mel liegt narzißt Identif mit dem Objekt zu Grunde. Die Differenzen liegen darin, daß die Dem unzweifelhaft früher auftritt als die Par, obwol ihre lib. Disposition weiter zurückreicht und daß MelManie keine sichere zeitliche Einreihg gestatten. Man kann es also nicht festhalten, daß die sicher vorhanden

10 die fast unausweichlich [illegible] die frühesten. Es spielte die Konv.hy (neu zu G. [illegible]) an. noch etwas später in der Hauptperiode (9–10) weit bei Kindern die Zw. auch die narzisst. Neurosen folgen das Kindheit. Von diesen ist die Dem. pr. in der klassischen Form Erkrankung der Pubertätsjahre, die Paranoia nähert sich den Jahren der Reife, und Mel-Manie auch demselben Zeitabschnitt, sonst unbestimmbar. Die Reihe lautet also:

Angsthy – Konv.hy – Zw.Neur. – Dem. pr. – Paranoia – Mel-Manie

Die Fixierungsdispositionen dieser Affektionen scheinen auch eine Reihe zu ergeben, die aber gegenläufig ist. ~~Deutlich~~ bes. wenn man bed. Dispositionen vornehmlich, so ergibt sich also, je später die Neurose auftritt, auf desto früherer Libidophase muss sie regredieren. Dies gilt indess nur im grossen Ganzen. Unzweifelhaft richtig [illegible] Angsthy gegen Konv. [illegible] die Zw. gegen die [illegible] Vorstufen der 3 Übertragungsneurosen gegen vollzogene Libidoentwicklung. Die narzisst. Neurosen aber gehen auf Phasen vor der Objektfindung zurück, die Dem. pr. regrediert bis zum Autoerotismus, die Paranoia bis zur narzisst. homosex. Objektwahl, die Mel. liegt wahrscheinlich mit dem Objekt zu Grunde. Die Differenzen liegen darin, dass die Dem. [illegible] früher auftritt als die Par., obwohl ihre Disposition weiter zurückreicht, und dass Mel. Manie keine [illegible] Einreihung gestatten. Man kann es also nicht festhalten, dass die früher verfallenen

11 Zeitreihe der ΨN allein durch die Libentwicklg bestim̄t wäre. Soweit dies zutrifft würde man die umgekehrte Beziehg zwischen beiden betonen. Es ist auch bekannt daß mit Altersfortschritt Hy oder Zw in Dem sich umsetzen kann, nie kom̄t das Umgekehrte vor.

Man kann aber eine andere phylogenet. Reihe aufstellen, die wirklich mit der Zeitreihe der Neuros gleichläufig ist. Nur muß man dabei weit ausholen u sich manches hypothetische Zwischenglied gefallen laßen.

Von Dr Wittels ist zuerst die Idee ausgesprochen worden, daß das Urmenschentier seine Existenz in einem überaus reichen, alle Bedürfniße befriedigenden Milieu hingebracht, dessen Nachhall wir im Mythus vom uranfänglichen Paradies erhalten haben. Dort mag es die Periodizität der Libido überwunden haben, die den Säugetieren noch anhaftet. Ferenczi hat dann in der bereits erwähnten gedankenreichen Arbeit die Idee ausgesprochen, daß die weitere Entwicklg dieses Urmenschen unter dem Einfluß der geologischen Erdschicksale erfolgt ist, und daß insbesondere die Not der Eiszeiten ihm die Anregung zur Kulturentwicklg gebracht hat. Es wird ja allgemein zugegeben, daß die Menschenart zur Eiszeit bereits bestand und ihre Einwirkg an sich erfahren hat.

Greifen wir die Idee von Ferenczi auf, so liegt die Versuchung sehr nahe, in den 3 Dispositionen zur Angsthy, Konversionshy und Zwangs Regressionen auf Phasen zu ~~sehen,~~ erkennen, welche

11 Zeitreihe der ÜN allein durch die Libidoentwicklg bestimmt wäre. Soweit aber das entscheidende Moment die Ichgegensätze beider betrifft, zu erkennen. Es ist auch bekannt, daß mit Altersfortschritt Hy oder ZN zu Dem sich umwandeln kann, wie dann des Ausgangsbild war.

Man kann aber eine andere zusammengehörige Reihe aufstellen, die wirklich mit der Zeitreihe der Neurosen gleichläufig ist und nun muß man daran gehen, sich manches phylogenetische Zweifelhafte gefallen lassen.

Von Dr Wittels ist zuerst die Idee ausgesprochen worden, daß das Menschentier seine Existenz in einem überaus reichen, alle Bedürfnisse befriedigenden Milieu hingebracht hat, dessen Nachhall wir im Mythos vom urzeitlichen Paradies erhalten haben. Dort mag es die Periodizität der Libido überwunden haben, die den Säugetieren noch anhaftet. Ferenczi hat dann in der an bemerkenswerten Gedankenreichen Arbeit die Idee ausgesprochen, daß die weitere Entwicklung dieses Urmenschen unter dem Einfluß der geologischen Erdschicksale erfolgt ist, und daß speziell die Not der Eiszeiten ihm die Anregung zur Kulturentwicklung gebracht hat. Es wird ja allgemein zugegeben, daß die Menschenart zur Eiszeit bereits bestand und ihre Einwirkung an sich erfahren hat.

Greifen wir die Idee von Ferenczi auf, so liegt die Versuchung sehr nahe, in den 3 Dispositionen zu Angsthy, Konversionshy und Zwangsneurosen auf Regressionen ~~zu sehen~~, erkennen zu wollen

12 dereinst die ganze Menschenart vom Beginne bis zum Ende der Eiszeiten durchzumachen hatte, so daß damals alle Menschen so waren wie heute nur ein Anteil kraft seiner erblichen Veranlagung und durch Neuerwerbung ist. Die Bilder können sich natürlich nicht völlig decken, denn die Neurose enthält mehr als was die Regression mit sich bringt. Sie ist auch der Ausdruck des Sträubens gegen diese Regression und ein Kompromiß zwischen dem urzeitlich Alten und dem Anspruch des kulturell Neuen. Am stärksten wird sich diese Differenz bei der Zwneurose ausprägen müßen, welche wie keine andere unter dem Zeichen der inneren Gegensätzlichkeit steht. Doch muß die Neurose, soweit das Verdrängte in ihr. gesiegt hat, das urzeitliche Bild wiederbringen.

Unsere erste Aufstellung würde also behaupten, daß die Menschheit unter dem Einfluß der Entbehrungen, welche ihr die hereinbrechende Eiszeit auferlegte allgemein ängstlich geworden ist. Die bisher vorwiegend freundliche, jede Befriedigg spendende Außenwelt verwandelte sich in eine Haufung von drohenden Gefahren. Es war aller Grund zur Realangst vor allem Neuen gegeben. Die sex Libido verlor allerdings zunächst ihre Objekte, die ja menschliche sind, nicht, aber es läßt sich denken, daß das in seiner Existenz bedrohte Ich von der Objektbesetzung

12 durchlebt die ganze Menschheit vom Beginne bis zum Ende der Eiszeit durchzumachen hatte, so daß damals alle Menschen so wurden wie heute nur ein Anteil durch seine erbliche Veranlagung und durch Neuerwerbung ist also [illegible] keineswegs natürlich nicht völlig [illegible], denn die [illegible] entfällt durch als was die Regression mit sich bringt. Sie ist auch der Ausdruck des Sträubens gegen diese Regression und ein Kompromiss zwischen dem möglichst [illegible] und dem Anspruch des Kulturmenschen. Am stärksten wird sich diese Differenz bei der Zwangsneurose ausprägen müssen, welche wie schon erwähnt unter dem Einfluß der inneren Gegensätzlichkeit durchaus nicht die Neurose, sowie das Verdrängte [illegible] hat das möglichst viel beizubringen.

Unsere erste Aufstellung würde also behaupten, daß die Menschheit unter dem Einfluß der Entbehrungen, welche ihr das hereinbrechende Eiszeitalter auferlegte, allgemein ängstlich geworden ist. Die bisher vorwiegend freundliche, jede Befriedigung spendende Außenwelt verwandelte sich in eine Häufung von drohenden Gefahren. Es war aller Grund zur Realangst vor allem Neuen gegeben. Die sexuelle Libido verlor allerdings zunächst ihre Objekte, die ja menschlich sind, nicht, aber es läßt sich denken, daß das in seiner Existenz bedrohte Ich von der Objektbesetzung

13 einigermaßen absah ~~und~~ die Libido im Ich erhielt und so in Realangst verwandelte, was vorher Objektlibido gewesen war. An der infantilen Angst sehen wir nun, daß das Kind die Objektlibido im Falle der Unbefriedigg in Realangst vor dem Fremden verwandelt, aber auch, daß es übhpt dazu neigt, sich vor allem Neuen zu ängstigen. Wir haben einen langen Streit darüber geführt, ob die Realangst oder die Sehnsuchtangst das ursprünglichere ist, ob das Kind seine Libido in Realangst wandelt, weil es für zu groß, gefährlich erachtet u so übhpt zur Vorstellg der Gefahr kom̅t, oder ob es vielmehr einer allgemeinen Ängstlichkeit nachgiebt und aus dieser lernt, sich auch vor seiner unbefriedigten Libido zu fürchten. Unsere Neigung gieng dahin das erstere anzunehmen, die Sehnsuchtangst voranzustellen, aber dazu fehlte uns eine besondere Disposition. Wir mußten es für eine allgemein-kindliche Neigung erklären. Die phylogenetische Uberlegung scheint nun diesen Streit zu Gunsten der Realangst zu schlichten u läßt uns annehmen, daß ein Anteil der Kinder die Angstlichkeit des Beginns der Eiszeiten mitbringt und nun durch sie verleitet wird die unbefriedigte Libido wie eine außere Gefahr zu behandeln. Das relative Ubermaß der Libido würde aber derselben Anlage entspringen u die Neuerwerbung der disponirten Ängstlichkeit ermöglichen. Im̅erhin würde die Diskussion der Angsthysterie das Ubergewicht

13 eingeschränkten [illegible] die Libido in Ich-[illegible] und so in Realangst verwandelt, was vorher Objektlibido gewesen war.

An der infantilen Angst haben wir gemeint, dass das Kind die Objektlibido im Falle der Unbefriedigung in Realangst vor dem Fremden verwandelt, aber auch dass es überhaupt dazu neigt, sich vor allem Neuen zu ängstigen. Wir haben einen langen Streit darüber geführt, ob die Realangst oder die Sehnsuchtsangst das ursprünglichere ist, ob das Kind seine Libido in Realangst wandelt, weil es sie für zu groß, gefährlich erachtet u. so überhaupt zur Vorstellung der Gefahr kommt, oder ob es vielmehr einer allgemeinen Ängstlichkeit nachgibt und von dieser lernt, sich auch vor seiner unbefriedigten Libido zu fürchten. Wir waren geneigt, das erstere anzunehmen, die Sehnsuchtangst voranzustellen, aber dazu fehlte uns eine besondere Disposition. Wir mussten es für eine allgemein-kindliche Neigung erklären. Die phylogenetische Betrachtung scheint nun diesen Streit zu Gunsten der Realangst zu schlichten u. läßt uns annehmen, dass ein Anteil der Kinder die Ängstlichkeit des Beginns der Eiszeit mitbringt und nun durch sie verleitet wird, die unbefriedigte Libido wie eine äußere Gefahr zu behandeln. Das relative Übermaß der Libido würde aber derselben Anlage entspringen u. die Neuerwerbung der [illegible] Ängstlichkeit ermöglichen. [illegible] würde die [illegible] der Angsthysterie das Übergewicht

14 der phylogenetischen Disposition über alle anderen Momente befürworten.

2). Mit dem Fortschritt der harten Zeiten mußte sich den in ihrer Existenz bedrohten Urmenschen der Konflikt zwischen Selbsterhaltung und Fortpflanzungslust ergeben, welcher in den meisten Fällen typischen von Hysterie seinen Ausdruck findet. Die Nahrungsmittel reichten nicht hin, eine Vermehrung der menschlichen Horden zu gestatten und die Kräfte des Einzelnen reichten nicht aus, soviele der Hilflosen am Leben zu erhalten. Die Tödtung der Geborenen fand sicherlich einen Widerstand an der Liebe besonders der Mütter narzißtischen. Somit wurde es soziale Pflicht, die Fortpflanzung zu beschränken. Die perversen nicht zur Kinderzeugg führenden Befriediggen entgiengen diesem Verbot, was eine gewiße Regression auf die Libidophase vor dem Primat der Genitalien beförderte. Die Einschränkg mußte das Weib härter treffen Abstinenz als den um die Folgen des Sexualverkehrs eher unbekümmerten Mann. Diese ganze Situation entspricht offenkundig den Bedinggen der Konversionshysterie. Aus der Symptomatik derselben schließen wir, daß der Mensch noch sprachlos war, als er sich aus der unbezwungenen Not das Verbot der Fortpflanzung auferlegte, also auch noch nicht das System des Vbw über seinem Ubw aufgebaut hatte. Auf die Konversshy regredirt dann auch der dazu Disponirte, speziell das Weib

14 der phylogenetischen Disposition aller
andern Neurosen befunden worden.
2. Mit dem Fortschritt der harten Zeiten
mußte sich den von Eiszeit bedrohten
Menschen der Konflikt zwischen Selbsterhaltung und Fortpflanzungslust ergeben,
welcher in den meisten typischen Fällen
von Hysterie seinen Ausdruck findet.
Die Nahrungsmittel reichten nicht hin,
um eine Vermehrung der menschlichen Horden
zu gestatten und die Kräfte des Einzelnen
reichten nicht aus, so viele Hilflose am
Leben zu erhalten. Die Tötung der Neugebore-
nen fand sicherlich einen Widerstand an der
Liebe, besonders der narzißtischen
Mütter. So wurde es soziale Pflicht, die Fortpflanzung zu beschränken. Die perversen
nicht zur Kinderzeugung führenden Befrie-
digungen entgingen diesem Verbot, was
eine gewisse Regression auf die Libidophase vor dem Primat der Genitalien
beförderte. Die Einschränkung (Abstinenz) wirkte auf das
Weib härter als auf den Mann, der die
Folgen des Sexualverkehrs eher unbe-
kümmerte. Diese ganze Situation
entspricht offenkundig den Bedingungen
der Konversionshysterie. Aus der Symptomatik derselben schließen wir, daß der
Mensch noch sprachlos war, als er sich aus
der Notwendigkeit, nicht das Verbot
der Fortpflanzung auferlegte, also
auch noch nicht das System des Vbw
über seinem Ubw aufgebaut hatte.
Auf die Konversionshy. regrediert dann auch
das dazu disponierte, speziell das Weib

15 unter dem Einfluß der Verbote, welche die Genitalfunktion ausschalten wollen, während stark erregende frühzeitige Eindrücke zur Genitalbetätigg drängen.

3). Die weitere Entwicklg ist leicht zu konstruiren. Sie betraf vorwiegend den Mann. Nachdem er gelernt hatte an der Libido zu sparen und die Sexualtätigkeit durch Regression auf eine frühere Phase zu erniedrigen, gewann die Betatigg der Intelligenz für ihn die Hauptrolle. Er lernte forschen, die Welt feindliche etwas verstehen und sich durch Erfindungen eine erste Herrschaft über sie zu sichern. Er entwickelte sich unter dem Zeichen der Energie, bildete die Anfänge der Sprache aus u mußte den Neuerwerbungen große Bedeutg zulegen. Die Sprache war ihm Zauber, seine Gedanken erschienen ihm allmächtig, er verstand die Welt nach seinem Ich. Es ist die Zeit der animistischen Weltanschauung u ihrer magischen Technik. Zum Lohn für seine Kraft, so vielen anderen hilflosen Lebenssicherung zu schaffen, maßte er sich die uneingeschränkte Herrschaft über sie an, vertrat durch seine Persönlichkeit die beiden ersten Setzungen, daß er selbst unverletzlich sei und daß ihm die Verfügung über die Frauen nicht bestritten werden dürfe. Zu Ende dieses Zeitabschnitts war das Menschengeschlecht in einzelne Horden zerfallen, die von einem starken und weisen brutalen Mann als Vater beherrscht wurden. Es ist möglich, daß die egoistisch eifersüchtige u rücksichtslose Natur, die wir nach völkerpsychologischen Erwäggen dem Urvater der Menschenhorde zuschreiben

15 mehr zum Ausdruck des Verbots, welche die
Gestaltfunktion ausschalten wollen, während
stark vorwiegend gleichzeitige Eindrücke
zur Gestaltbildung drängen.
3). Die weitere Entwicklung ist leicht zu konstruieren.
Der Antrieb [illegible] den Menschen so
[illegible] hatte, den der Liebe zu [illegible] und
die [illegible] durch [illegible]
[illegible] zu [illegible], gewann
die [illegible] die Intelligenz für ihn die
Herrschaft. Er lernte [illegible], die Welt
[illegible] zu verstehen und sich durch Erfindungen eine [illegible] Herrschaft über sie
zu sichern. Er entwickelte sich unter dem
[illegible] des [illegible] bildete die [illegible]
der Sprache aus und machte den [illegible]
[illegible] großen [illegible] Die Sprache
war ihm Zauber [illegible] Gedanken [illegible]
ihm allmächtig zu [illegible] die Welt
nach seinem [illegible] die [illegible]
[illegible] Weltanschauung [illegible] magischer
Zeitalter. [illegible]
[illegible] Lebensbedürfnis-
[illegible]
[illegible] über [illegible]
[illegible] die beiden
[illegible]
[illegible] ihm die [illegible] über
[illegible] nicht [illegible] werden
[illegible]
[illegible] in [illegible]
[illegible] und
[illegible] Vater [illegible]
[illegible] werden. Es ist möglich, daß die [illegible]
[illegible] hatten die
[illegible] psychologischen Ereignissen
[illegible] der Menschheit [illegible]

wichtig

16 nicht von Anfang an vorhanden war, sondern sich im Laufe der schweren Eiszeiten als Resultat der Anpassung an die Not herausgebildet hat.

Die Charaktere dieser Menschheitsphase wiederholt nun die ~~Menschheitsp~~ Zwangsneurose, einen Teil derselben negativ, da ja die Neurose dem Sträuben gegen Reaktionsbildgen diese Wiederkehr mitentspricht. Die Überbetonung des Denkens, die riesige Energie, die ~~als~~ im Zwang wiederkehrt, die Allmacht der Gedanken, sind unverwandelte Züge. Aber gegen die brutalen Impulse, welche das Liebesleben ersetzen wollen, erhebt sich der Widerstand späterer Entwicklungen die Neigung zu unverbrüchlichen Gesetzen, der von dem libidinösen Konflikt aus endlich die Lebensenergie des Individuums lähmt und nur die auf Geringfugiges verschobenen Impulse als Zwang bestehen läßt, übrig. So geht dieser für die Kulturentwicklg wertvollste menschliche Typus an den Ansprüchen des Liebeslebens zu Grunde in seiner Wiederkehr, wie der großartige Typus des Urvaters selbst, der später als Gottheit wiederkehrte, an den familiären Verhältnißen, die er sich schuf, in der Wirklichkeit zu Grunde gegangen ist.

4). Soweit wären wir in der Erfüllg eines von Ferenczi vorhergesehenen Programs »die neurotischen Regressionstypen mit den Etappen der Stamesgeschichte der Menschheit in Einklang zu bringen« gekomen, vielleicht ohne in allzu gewagte Spekulationen abzuirren. Für die weiteren und später

16 nicht von Anfang an vorhanden war, sondern
sich mit Aufhebung des früheren Zustandes als
Reaktion der Anpassung an die Not herausgebildet hat.
Die Charaktere dieser Menschheitsphase
wiederholt nun die ~~Menschheits~~ Zwangsneurose, zum Teil derselben reaktiv das
[illegible] dem Streben gegen
[illegible] wiederkehrt, unverkennbar die Überbetonung des Denkens, die riesige Energie,
die im Zwang wiederkehrt, die Allmacht
der Gedanken, und [illegible]
(Hyp.) etwa gegen die brutalen Impulse
welche das Liebesleben ersetzen wollen,
erhebt sich der Widerstand späterer Entwicklungen, der Neigung zu unverbrüchlichen Gesetzen, der von dem Liebesleben
[illegible]
[illegible]
[illegible] Zwang [illegible]
[illegible] Lebens [illegible]
[illegible]
[illegible]
[illegible]
[illegible]
[illegible]
[illegible]
[illegible]
III. [illegible]
[illegible]
[illegible]
[illegible]
[illegible]
[illegible]
[illegible]

17 auftretenden narzißtischen Neurosen fehlte uns aber jede Anknüpfg, wenn uns nicht die Annahme zu Hilfe käme, daß die Disposition zu ihnen von einer zweiten Generation erworben worden ist, deren Entwicklg in eine neue Phase menschlicher Kultur hinüberleitet.

Diese zweite Generation hebt mit den Söhnen an welchen der eifersüchtige Urvater nicht gewähren läßt. Wir haben an anderer Stelle (T u T) eingesetzt, daß er sie vertreibt, wenn sie das Alter der Pubertät erreicht haben. ΨA Erfahrungen mahnen aber eine andere u grausamere Lösung an die Stelle zu setzen, nämlich daß er sie ihrer Mannheit beraubt, wonach sie als unschädliche Hilfsarbeiter in der Horde bleiben können.

Den Effekt der Kastration in jener Urzeit dürfen wir uns wol als Erlöschen der Libido und Stehenbleiben in der indiv Entwicklg vorstellen. Solchen Zustand scheint die Dem pr. zu wiederholen, die zumal als Hebephrenie zum Aufgeben jedes Liebesobjekts, Rückbildg aller Sublimirungen und Rückkehr zum Autoerotismus führt. ~~Was~~ Das jugendliche Individ verhält sich so, als ob es die Kastration erlitten hätte; ja ~~Selb~~ wirkliche Selbstkastrationen sind bei dieser Affektion nicht selten. Was die Krankheit sonst auszeichnet, die Sprachverändergen, u halluzinat Stürme darf man in das phylogenet. Bild nicht einbeziehen, denn sie entsprechen den Heilungsversuchen, den vielfältigen Bemühungen, das Objekt wiederzugewin̄en, die im Krankheitsbilde beinahe auffälliger
Zeitlang. sind als die Rückbildgserscheinungen.

17 entstandenen narzißtischen Neurosen fehlt
uns aber jede Erkenntnis ferne und
nur die Annahme zu Hilfe kommen, daß
die Disposition zu ihnen von einer zweiten
Generation erworben worden ist, deren
Entwicklung in eine neue Phase menschlicher Kultur hinüberleitet [?].
Diese zweite Generation hebt mit den Söhnen
an, welchen der eifersüchtige Vater
nicht gewähren läßt. Wir haben an anderer
Stelle (T. u. T.) ausgeführt, daß er sie vertreibt,
wenn sie das Alter der Pubertät erreicht
haben. Die ψa Erfahrungen mahnen aber eine
andere u. grausamere Lösung an die Stelle
zu setzen, nämlich daß er sie ihrer Mannheit
beraubt, worauf sie als unschädliche Hilfsarbeiter in der Horde bleiben konnten.
Den Effekt der Kastration in jener Urzeit dürfen
wir uns wol als Erlöschen der Libido und
Stehenbleiben in der indiv. Entwicklung vorstellen. Solchen Zustand scheint die Dem. pr.
zu wiederholen, die zumal als Adolescenz [?]
zum Aufgeben jedes Liebesobjekts, Rück-
bildung aller Sublimierungen und Rückkehr
zum Autoerotismus führt. ~~Wie~~ Das jugendliche Individuum verhält sich, als ob es die
Kastration erlitten hätte; ja ~~volle~~ wirkliche Selbstkastrationen sind bei diesen
Affektion nicht selten. Was die Krankheit
sonst auszeichnet, die Sprachveränderungen
und halluzinat. Stürme, darf man in
die Symptome nicht einbeziehen.
Denn sie entsprechen den Heilungsversuchen, den vielfältigen Bemühungen
das Objekt wiederzugewinnen, die
im Krankheitsbild meist überwiegen [?]
Zeitlang. nur als die Krankheitserscheinungen.

18 Mit der Annahme einer solchen Behandlg der Söhne hängt eine Frage zusam̄en, die im Vorübergehen zu beantworten ist. Woher kom̄t den Urvätern Nachfolge und Ersatz, wenn sie sich der Söhne in solcher Weise entledigen. Schon Atkinson hat den Weg gewiesen, indem er hervorhob, daß nur die älteren Söhne die volle Verfolgg des Vaters zu befürchten hatten, daß aber der jüngste – schematisch gedacht – ~~wel~~ dank der Furbitte der Mutter vor allem aber infolge des Alterns ~~und de~~ des Vaters u seiner Hilfsbedürfigkeit Aussicht hatte, diesem Schicksal zu entgehen und der Nachfolger des Vaters zu werden. Dieser Vorzug des Jüngsten wurde in der nächstkom̄enden sozialen Gestaltung gründlich beseitigt und durch das Vorrecht des Altesten ersetzt. Im Mythus u im Märchen ist er aber sehr gut kenntlich erhalten.

5). Die nächste Wandlg konnte nur darin bestehen, daß die bedrohten Söhne sich der Kastration durch die Flucht entzogen und lernten mit einander verbündet den Kampf des Lebens auf sich zu nehmen. Dies Zusam̄enleben mußte sozialen Gefüle zeitigen und konnte auf homosexueller Sexualbefriedigg aufgebaut sein. Es ist sehr möglich, daß in der Vererbung dieser Zustandsphase die lange gesuchte hered. Disposition der Homosexualität zu erblicken ist. Die hier entstandenen aus der Homosex sublimirten sozialen Gefüle wurden aber zum dauernden Menschheitsbesitz und zur Grundlage jeder späteren Gesellschaft. Diese Zustandsphase bringt aber

18 Mit der Annahme einer solchen Beschaffenheit der Söhne steigt eine Frage auf, die zu [illegible] zu beantworten ist. Woher kamen dann die Nachfolger und Ersatz, wenn sie sich der Söhne in solcher Weise entledigten. Schon Atkinson hat den Weg gewiesen, indem er hervorhob, daß nur die älteren Söhne die volle Verfolgung des Vaters zu befürchten haben, daß aber der jüngste – schematisch gedacht – dank der Fürsprache der Mutter vor allem aber infolge des Alterns und der des Vaters Hilfsbedürftigkeit Aussicht hatte, diesem Schicksal zu entgehen und der Nachfolger des Vaters zu werden. Diese Bevorzugung des Jüngsten wurde in der nächstfolgenden sozialen Gestaltung gründlich beseitigt und durch das Vorrecht des Ältesten ersetzt. Im Mythus und Märchen ist es aber noch gut kenntlich erhalten.

5) Die nächste Wandlung konnte nur darin bestehen, daß die bedrohten Söhne sich der Kastration durch die Flucht entzogen und verbündet miteinander den Kampf ums Leben auf sich zu nehmen lernten. Dies Zusammenleben mußte die sozialen Gefühle zeitigen und konnte auf homosexueller Sexualbefriedigung aufgebaut sein. Es ist sehr möglich, daß in der Vererbung dieser Entwicklungsphase die lang gesuchte hered. Disposition der Homosexualität zu erblicken ist. Die hier entstandenen aus der homosexuellen Sublimierung sozialen Gefühle wurden zum dauernden Menschheitsbesitz und zur Grundlage jeder späteren Gesellschaft. Diese Entwicklungsphase bringt aber

19 ersichtlich die Par wieder; richtiger gegen die Wiederkehr ders. wehrt sich die Par, bei der die geheimen Bündniße nicht fehlen und der Verfolger eine großartige Rolle spielt. Die Par. sucht die Homosex. abzuwehren, welche die Grundlage der Brüderorganisation war, und muß dabei den Befallenen aus der Gesellschaft treiben, seine sozialen Sublimirgen zerstören und.

6). Die Einreihung der Mel-Manie in diesen Zusam̄enhang scheint auf die Schwierigkeit zu stoßen, daß eine Normalzeit für das individuelle Auftreten dieses neurotischen Leidens nicht sicher anzugeben ist. Doch steht es fest, daß sie eher dem Alter der Reife angehört als der Kindheit faßt die man charakterist. Abwechslung von Depression und Hochstim̄ung ins Auge, so ist es schwer sich an nicht die so ähnliche Aufeinanderfolge von Triumph und Trauer zu erinnern, welche regelmäßigen Bestand religiöser Festlichkeiten bildet. Trauer über den Tod des Gottes, Triumphfreude über seine Wiederaufstehung. Dieses religiöse Zeremoniell wiederholt aber nur, wie wir aus den Angaben der Völkerpsychologie erraten haben, in umkehrender Richtung das Verhalten der Mitglieder des Brüderklans, nachdem sie den Urvater über~~fallen~~ wältigt und getödtet hatten: Triumph über seinen Tod und dann Trauer darüber, da sie ihn doch alle als. Vorbild verehrt hatten. So gäbe dieses große Ereignis der Menschengeschichte welches der Urhorde ein Ende machte

19 verpflichtet die Par. werden, richtiger gegen
die Wiederkehr derer wehrt sich die Par.,
bei der die geheimen Bündnisse nicht fehlen
und der Verfolger eine großartige
Rolle spielt. Die Par. sucht die Homosexualität abzuwehren, welche die Grundlage der
Brüderorganisation war, und muss
dabei den Befallenen aus der
Gesellschaft treiben, seine sozialen
Sublimierungen zerstören.

Die Einreihung der Mel.-Manie in diese
6). Zusammenhang scheint auf die Schwierigkeit zu stoßen, daß eine Normalzeit
für das individuelle Auftreten dieses
neurotischen Leidens nicht anzugeben
ist. Doch steht es fest, daß sie eher dem Alter
der Reife angehört als der Kindheit.
Faßt man die charakteristische Abwechslung
von Depression und Hochstimmung ins Auge,
so ist es schwer, nicht an die so ähnliche
Aufeinanderfolge von Triumph und
Trauer zu erinnern, welche regelmäßigen
Bestand religiöser Festlichkeiten bildet.
Trauer über den Tod des Gottes, Triumphfreude über seine Wiederauferstehung.
Dieses religiöse Zeremoniell wiederholt
aber, wie wir aus den Angaben
der Völkerpsychologie erraten haben,
in umgekehrter Richtung das Verhalten der Mitglieder des Brüder-
clans, nachdem sie den Urvater über-
~~hatten~~ wältigt und getötet hatten:
Triumph über seinen Tod und dann
Trauer darüber, daß sie ihn doch alle
St./ Vorbild verehrt hatten. So gäbe dieses
große Ereignis der Menschheitsgeschichte
welches der Urhorde ein Ende machte

20 und sie durch die siegreiche Brüderorganisation ersetzte, die Praedisposition für die eigentümliche Stim̄ungsfolge, die wir als besondere narzißtische Affektion neben den Paraphrenien anerkennen.

Die Trauer ~~über~~ um den Urvater geht aus der Identifizirung mit ihm vor, und solche Identifizirg haben wir als die Bedingung des melancholischen Mechanismus nachgewiesen.

Zusam̄enfassend können wir sagen. Wenn die Dispositionen zu den 3 Ubertraggsneurosen im Kampf mit der Not der Eiszeiten erworben wurden, so stam̄en die Fixirungen, welche den narzißtischen Neurosen zu Grunde liegen aus der Bedrangung durch den Vater, welcher nach Ablauf der Eiszeit deren Rolle gleichsam gegen die zweite Generation übernim̄t, fortsetzt. Wie der erste Kampf zur patriarchalischen Kulturstufe führt, so der zweite zur sozialen, aber aus beiden ergeben sich die Fixirungen, die in ihrer Wiederkehr nach Jahrtausenden zur Disposition der zwei Gruppen von Neurosen werden. Auch in diesem Sinne ist also die Neurose ein Kulturerwerb

Ob die hier entworfene Parallele mehr ist als eine spielerische Vergleichung, in welchem Maße sie die noch nicht gelösten Rätsel der Neurosen zu beleuchten mag, darf füglich ferneren Untersuchungen und der Beleuchtg durch neue Erfahrungen überlassen werden ——

20 und sie durch die hysterische Verdrängung
[illegible] ersetzt. Die Prädisposition für
die eigentümliche Wirkungsweise, ein mit
als besondere narzisstische Affektion
neben der Dementia praecox anerkennen
die Frage über den Charakter geht aus dass
Identifizierung mit ihm, [illegible] und solche
Identifizierung klar, weil als die Bedingung
des melancholischen Mechanismus nach-
zuweisen.

Zusammenfassend können wir sagen. Wenn
die Dispositionen zu den 3 Übertragungsneurosen im Kampf mit der Not der
Eiszeiten erworben wurden, so [illegible]
die Fixierungen, welche den narzisstischen
Neurosen zu Grunde liegen aus der
Bedrängung durch den Vater, welcher
nach Ablauf der Eiszeit diese Rolle
gleichsam gegen die zweite Generation über-
nimmt, fortsetzt. Wie der erste Kampf
zur patriarchalischen Kulturstufe führt
der zweite zur sozialen, aber aus beiden
ergeben sich die Fixierungen, die in ihrer
Wiederkehr nach Jahrtausenden zur
Disposition der zwei Gruppen von Neurosen
werden. Auch in diesem Sinne ist also
die Neurose ein Kulturerwerb.

Ob die hier entworfene Parallele
mehr ist als eine spielerische Vergleichung, in welchem Maße sie die
noch ungelösten Rätsel der Neurosen
zu beleuchten vermag, darf füglich
ferneren Untersuchungen und der
Beleuchtung durch neue Erfahrungen
überlassen werden.

21 Nun ist Zeit Reihe Einwendungen zu denken, die mahnen, daß wir die erreichten Zurückführgen nicht uberschatzen sollen. Zunächst jedem aufdrängen, daß die zweite Reihe der Dispositionen, die der zweiten Generation, nur von Männern (als Söhnen) erworb werden konnten, während Dem pr, Paran u Mel ebensowol von Frauen produzirt werden. Frauen in Urzeiten unter noch mehr verschiedenen Bedingg gelebt als heute. Sodann haftet an diesen Dispositionen eine Schwierigkeit, von der die ersten Reihe frei sind: Sie scheinen unter Bedinggen erworb zu werden, die Vererbung ausschließen. Es ist evident, daß die kastrirten u eingeschüchterten Söhne nicht zur Fortpflanzg kom̄en, also ihre Disposition nicht fortsetzen können (Dem pr). Aber ebensowenig kann der ψ Zustand der ausgetriebenen in Homosex verbundenen Söhne Einfluß auf die nächsten Generationen nehmen da sie als unfruchtbare Seitenzweige der Familie erlöschen, so lange sie nicht über den Vater triumphirt haben. Bringen sie es aber zu diesem Triumph, so ist es Erlebnis einer Generation, dem man die notwendige unbegrenzte Vervielfältigg absprechen muß. ~~Wie~~

Wie sich denken läßt, braucht man auf so dunkeln Gebieten um Auskünfte nicht verlegen zu sein. Die Schwierigkeit fällt ja im Grunde mit einer früher aufgeworf- ~~zu St~~ zusam̄en, wie sich der brutale Vater der Eiszeit, der ja nicht unsterblich war wie sein göttliches Nachbild, fortgesetzt. Wieder bietet sich der jüngere Sohn, der später zum Vater wird, der zwar nicht selbst kastrirt wird, aber das Schicksal seiner älteren

21 [illegible] ist Zeit, [illegible] Einwendungen zu denken, die mahnen daß wir die erreichten Wahrscheinlichkeiten nicht überschätzen sollen. Zunächst [illegible] aufdrängen, daß die zweite Reihe der Dispositionen, die der zweiten Generation, nur von den Männern (als Söhnen) erworben werden konnten, während Dem. pr., Paranoia u. Mel. ebensowol von Frauen [illegible] werden. Frauen in Urzeiten [illegible] sehr verschiedenen Bedingungen [illegible] als heute. [illegible]

[illegible]

22 Brüder kennt u für sich befürchtet, an den die Versuchung herangetreten sein muß wie die glucklicheren von ihnen zu fliehen u auf das Weib zu verzichten. So bliebe neben den als unfruchtbar abfallenden Männern im̄er eine Kette von anderen, die an ihrer Person die Schicksale des Männergeschlechts durchmachen u als Dispositionen vererben können. Der wesentliche Gesichtspunkt bleibt bestehen, daß sich für ihn die Not der Zeiten durch den Druck des Vaters ersetzt.

Der Triumph über den Vater muß ungezälte Generationen hindurch geplant u phantasirt worden sein ehe es gelang ihn zu realisiren.

Die Ausbreitg der durch den Vaterdruck erzeugten Dispositionen auf das Weib scheint selbst großere Schwierigkeit zu bereiten. Die Schicksale des Weibes in diesen Urzeiten sind uns durch besonderes Dunkel verhüllt. So mögen Lebensverhaltniße in Betracht kom̄en, die wir nicht erkannt haben. Der gröbsten Schwierigkeit uberhebt uns aber die Bemerkg, daß wir der Bisexualit des Menschen nicht vergeßen dürfen. So kann das Weib die vom Mann erworb Dispositionen übernehmen und selbst an sich zum Vorschein bringen.

Indeß machen wir uns klar, daß wir mit diesen Auskünften im Grund nichts anderes erreicht als unsere wissensch. Phantasien dem Vorwurf der Absurdität entzogen zu haben. Im Ganzen behalten sie ihren Wert als heilsame Ernüchtergen, wenn wir vielleicht auf Wege waren, die phylogent. Disposition über alles andere zu setzen. Es geht also nicht so zu, daß in vielleicht gesetzmäßig festgestellter Verhältniszal archaiische

22 wurde demnach hier sich beschränkt an den die Verfolgung herausforderten, sehr nahe wie die glücklicheren Brüder-Horde zu flüchten u. auf das Weib zu verzichten. So blieben neben den als unfruchtbar abfallenden Männern immer eine Gattung von anderen, die an ihrer Person die Schicksale des Männergeschlechts durchmachen u. als Dispositionen vererben können. Der wesentliche Gesichtspunkt bleibt bestehen, daß sich hier ihr die Not der Zeiten durch den Druck des Vaters ersetzt.

[illegible] Zwang über den Vater auch angezeigte Generationen hindurch Gegensatz u. Phantasie worden sein, ehe es gelang ihn zu beseitigen. Die Ausbreitung des Drucks der Naturbedingungen erzeugten Dispositionen auf das Weib scheint bloß größere Schwierigkeit zu bereiten. Die Schicksale des Weibes in diesen Urzeiten sind uns durch besonderes Dunkel verhüllt. So mögen Lebensverhältnisse in Betracht kommen, die wir nicht erkannt haben. Die größten Schwierigkeiten erspart uns aber die Bemerkung, daß wir der Bisexualität des Menschen nicht vergessen dürfen. So kann das Weib die vom Manne erworbenen Dispositionen übernehmen und selbst an sich zum Vorschein bringen.

Indeß machen wir uns klar, daß wir mit diesen Ausführungen im Grunde nichts anderes erreicht als unsere wissenschaftl. Phantasien dem Vorwurf der Absurdität entzogen zu haben. Im Ganzen behalten sie ihren Wert als heilsame Ernüchterungen wenn wir vielleicht durch Drang waren die phylogenet. [illegible] über alles andere zu setzen. Es ist also nicht so zu [illegible], daß in vielleicht [illegible] gesetzmäßig festgestellten [illegible] [illegible]

23 Konstitution an den neuen Indiv wiederkehren und sie durch den Konflikt mit den Ansprüchen der Gegenwart in Neurose drängen. Es bleibt Raum für Neuerwerbg und für Einflüße, die wir nicht kennen. Im Ganzen sind wir nicht am Ende, sondern zu Anfang eines Verständnißes dieses phylogenet. Faktors.

23 ~~Beobachtungen an den~~ neuen Individuen [illegible]
und die [illegible] der [illegible] der [illegible]
der [illegible] im Menschen [illegible] sich alle
[illegible] und [illegible] die
nur noch [illegible]. Die Begriffe [illegible] nicht am
Ende, sondern zu Anfang eines Verständ-
nisses dieses Phänomens [illegible].

On the back of the last page of the manuscript ⟨the letter is translated in the Preface⟩:

28. 7. 15

Lieber Freund

Ich schicke Ihnen hier den Entwurf der XII, der Sie gewiß interessiren wird. Sie können ihn wegwerfen oder behalten. Die Reinschrift folgt ihm Satz für Satz u weicht nur wenig von ihm ab. Seite 21–23 sind nach Ihrem Brief hinzugefügt, auf den ich gewartet hatte. Ihr ausgezeichneter Einwand war zum Glück vorgesehen worden. Ich werde nun eine Pause eintreten lassen, ehe ich Bw u Angst endgiltig ausarbeite. Ich leide viel an Karlsbader Beschwerden.

Herzl Gruß Ihr Freud

Envelope (reduced) in which Freud sent the manuscript to Ferenczi

28. 7. 15

Lieber Freund

Ich schicke Ihnen hier den Entwurf des XII, der Sie gewiß interessieren wird. Sie können ihn wegwerfen oder behalten. Die Reinschrift folgt ihm Satz für Satz u weicht nur wenig von ihm ab. Seite 21–23 sind nach Ihrem Briefe hinzugefügt, auf den ich gewartet hatte. Ihr entgegenkommender Einwand war zum Glück vorhergesehen worden.

Ich werde nun mein [illegible] ruhen lassen, ehe ich Bw u Angst endgiltig ausarbeite. Ich leide viel an Karlsbader Beschwerden.

Herzl Gruß Ihr Freud

Eingeschrieben

Mrs Do
for Dr. Fe

Herrn Dr S. Ferenczi

R WIEN 66 № 721

Budapest
en

VII Erzsebet-körut 54

Wine = coups
Kühen

Metapsychology and Metabiology

On Sigmund Freud's Draft Overview of the Transference Neuroses

ILSE GRUBRICH-SIMITIS

A hitherto unknown text of Sigmund Freud from one of the most productive of his creative periods surely will immediately become the object of careful exegesis, even if we are here dealing only with the rough draft and not with the fully elaborated final version of the lost twelfth metapsychological paper of 1915. In order to facilitate understanding, a sketch of three overlapping contextual levels—the biographical context, the work context, and the historicoscientific context—accompanies this first publication of the manuscript.

The Biographical Context

World War I had already been under way for several months when, at the end of 1914, in letters to his coworkers and students, Freud first mentioned the series of metapsychological papers he had begun to write after completing his paper on narcissism (1914c) and the case history of the "Wolf-Man" (1918b [1914]). On November 25 he alluded to the project in a letter to Lou Andreas-Salomé: "I am working in private on certain matters which are wide in scope and also perhaps rich in content" (1966a [1912–36], p. 21). Barely a month later a letter to Karl Abraham contains a precise summary of the central themes of the metapsychology plan:

> I recently discovered a characteristic of both systems, the conscious (cs) and the unconscious (ucs), which makes both almost intelligible and, I think, provides a simple solution of the problem of the relationship of dementia praecox to reality. All the cathexes of things form the system ucs, while the system cs corresponds to the linking of these unconscious representations with the word representations by way of which they may achieve entry into consciousness. Repression in the transference neuroses consists in the withdrawal of the libido from the system cs, that

is, in the dissociation of the thing and word representations, while repression in the narcissistic neuroses consists in the withdrawal of libido from the unconscious thing representations, which is of course a far deeper disturbance. That is why dementia praecox changes language in the first instance, and on the whole treats word representations in the way in which hysteria treats thing representations, that is, it subjects them to the primary process with condensation, displacement and discharge.

Summarizing and anticipating the end result, Freud continues:

I might manage a theory of the neuroses with chapters on the vicissitudes of the instincts, repression and the unconscious if my working energy does not finally succumb to my depressed mood. (1965a, p. 206)

In fact, Freud believed that his productivity at this time was constantly being threatened by bad moods. His international connections were shrinking or were severed completely, and most of his colleagues had been inducted into the military. He admitted to Lou Andreas-Salomé that he felt "often . . . as alone as in the first ten years when I was surrounded by a desert; but I was younger then and still endowed with infinite energy and perseverance" (1966a [1912–36], p. 32). And in a letter to Ernest Jones dated December 25, 1914, he diagnoses, "I do not delude myself about the fact that the golden age of our science has been suddenly disrupted, that we are approaching a bad period and that it can only be a matter of keeping the fire glowing in individual hearths until a more favorable wind permits us to set it aflame again." In the same letter Freud complains about another reason for his bad mood, namely the drastic decline in his analytic practice: "As you can imagine, my medical activity has been reduced to a minimum, 2–3 hours daily . . . I tolerate this limitation actually least well, since I have been accustomed to ample work for twenty years and it is impossible for me to spend more than a fraction of my free time in productive activities."[1] Finally, he gives a third reason for his "bad temper." Faced with a dearth of new manuscripts, Freud worried about continuation of the psychoanalytic professional journals, the *Internationale Zeitschrift für ärztliche Psychoanalyse* and *Imago*: "Both depend for their

1. My thanks are due Sigmund Freud Copyrights Ltd., Colchester, England, for access to the transcription of this still partially unpublished letter. Orthography and punctuation have been carefully adapted to modern conventions, abbreviations for the most part have been written out in full, and editorial additions have been placed in square brackets. The same holds true for all subsequent quotations.

existence on the favour of a worthy but capricious publisher" (1966a [1912–36], p. 35). As he set out to write his series of metapsychological papers at the end of 1914, Freud was struggling so hard with the various causes of his bad mood that he stated, self-critically, "All these works suffer from the lack of good cheer in which I wrote them and from their function as a kind of sedative" (ibid.).

Although traces of these travails appear in most of his correspondence, they are nowhere more deeply etched than in the letters exchanged by Freud at that time with the Hungarian psychoanalyst Sándor Ferenczi. On July 31, 1915, shortly after sending Ferenczi his draft overview of the transference neuroses, Freud comments, "You are now really the only one who still works beside me." The extent to which Ferenczi, predestined by his manner of thinking and the requisite knowledge, became Freud's indispensable partner in discussion, especially in thinking through the phylogenetic part of the manuscript, can be demonstrated by excerpts from their still-unpublished correspondence, which is essential for understanding the recovered text.[2]

On the same day as the first-mentioned letter to Lou Andreas-Salomé, Freud remarks on his project to Ferenczi in a pleasurably secretive kind of way: something is "in process" which should not yet be talked about. "I only want to reveal to you that, on paths that have been trodden for a long time, I have finally found the solution to the riddle of time and space and the long-sought mechanism for the release of anxiety." A few days later, on December 2, 1914, he of course has to admit: "I have fared in this matter as the Germans have in the war. The first successes were surprisingly easy and great, and they thus tempted me to continue; but now I have arrived at such hard and impenetrable things that I am not sure of getting through." Nonetheless, as early as December 15, in the almost cheerful war imagery that seems somewhat strange to us today, he asserts with renewed confidence that the work is again going well.

I am living, as my brother says, in my private trench; I speculate and write, and after hard battles have got safely through the first line of riddles and difficulties. Anxiety, hysteria, and paranoia have capitulated. We shall see now how far the successes can be carried forward. A great many beautiful things have emerged in the process: the choice of neurosis, the regressions taken care of without a hitch.

2. I am indebted to Sigmund Freud Copyrights, Enid Balint of London, and Judith Dupont of Paris for permission to quote from the transcription of this correspondence. (A comparison of the wording with the original letters was not possible.)

At the beginning of 1915 Ferenczi invites Freud to visit him in Budapest for a "change of scene . . . in these oppressively hard times." Freud wires his refusal and explains in a letter dated January 11 that

> suddenly an eruption of ideas had appeared . . . after a long pause, and of such significant content that it was at first as though I had been blinded. It had to do with the metapsychology of consciousness, nothing less . . . When I approached it two days later, the rude awakening came. The thing resisted any depiction and presented such frightful gaps and difficulties that I broke off.

Then on February 18 Freud sends Ferenczi a "page about melancholia." This is evidently a sketch of the trains of thought later developed in "Mourning and Melancholia" (1917e [1915]), and on April 8 he writes: "I have finished . . . the second article of my synthetic series. It has to do with repression [1915d], the first with instincts and their vicissitudes [1915c]; my favourite will be the third, which deals with the unconscious [1915e]." As early as April 23 he reports:

> The series—Instincts, Repression, Unconscious—is now finished. The first piece already typeset by the *Zeitschrift* and in your hands, both of the others in the publisher's briefcase. The introduction, "Instincts," is not very enticing, to be sure, but the subsequent texts prove very fruitful. A fourth paper is needed, to compare the dream with dementia praecox;[3] it is also—already drafted. It goes with the metapsychology. The journal is now taken care of for a whole year, as far as I am concerned. *Vivant sequentes.*

Barely two months later, on June 21, Freud is able to report on a further extension of the series:

> Ten of the twelve papers are finished, two of them (Consciousness and Anxiety) of course in need of revision. I have just completed Conversion Hysteria; only Obsessional Neurosis and Synthesis of the Transference Neuroses are missing. There is much in it, but it has many peculiarities and is not properly completed.

In the letter of July 10 Freud can verify that now eleven of the twelve papers are finished—"or approximately so."

Two days later he elaborates for the first time on the twelfth paper. In order to permit comparison of the text of the letter with the draft, and to

3. This was "A Metapsychological Supplement to the Theory of Dreams" (1917d [1915]).

facilitate understanding of the subsequent discussion, this letter is reproduced here in its entirety:[4]

July 12, 1915

Dear Friend

In preparing next session's lectures on the transference neuroses[5] I am troubled by phantasies which are hardly suitable for public expression. So listen:

There is a series of chronological starting points in patients which runs thus:

Anxiety hysteria — conversion hysteria — obsessional neurosis — dementia praecox — paranoia — melancholia-mania.

Their libidinal predispositions run in general in the opposite direction: that is to say, the fixation lies with the former set in very late stages of development, with the latter in very early ones. That statement, however, is not faultless.

On the other hand this series seems to repeat phylogenetically an historical origin. What are now neuroses were once phases in human conditions.[6]

With the appearance of privations in the glacial period men became apprehensive: they had every reason for transforming libido into anxiety.

Having learned that propagation was now the enemy of self-preservation and must be restricted they became—still in the time before speech—hysterical.

After they developed speech and intelligence in the hard school of the glacial period they formed primal hordes under the two prohibitions of the primal father, their love-life having to remain egoistic and aggressive. Compulsion, as in the obsessional neurosis, struggled against any return to the former state. The neuroses that followed belong to the new epoch and were acquired by the sons.

To begin with they were forced to relinquish all sexual objects, or else they were robbed of all libido by being castrated: dementia praecox.

They then learned to organize themselves on a homosexual basis, being driven out by the father. The struggle against that signifies paranoia. Finally, they overpowered the father so as to effect an identification with him, triumphed over him and mourned him: mania-melancholia.

Your priority in all this is evident.

Freud.

4. It was, to be sure, previously published in the Freud biography by Ernest Jones (1957, p. 330), but in the context of a biased representation of Ferenczi's role in the collaboration at the time.

5. ⟨A more accurate translation of the original German would read, "In preparing the overview of the transference neuroses." Jones, apparently unaware that Freud was referring to the overview paper, assumed he was speaking of his forthcoming lectures on the subject.⟩

6. ⟨This phrase is perhaps best translated as "phases of the human condition." See note 40, p. 18.⟩

In his letter of reply three days later Ferenczi briefly addresses Freud's "wonderful linking together of *all* types of neuroses, all conceived of as phases in the development of mankind." But Ferenczi's response is too brief to satisfy Freud, because on July 18 he admonishes his friend that he "would have liked to have heard more critique about the phylogenetic fantasy." Ferenczi reacts promptly on July 24:

Your remark that you would like to have heard more of my critique about the plan of work that you call phylogenetic fantasy is justified. I was merely expressing my joy over the fact that my *ontogenetic* fantasies[7] so quickly received a phylogenetic sister. Even now I cannot say much more, but I find the analogy between the presumed phases in the development of mankind and[8] the neuroses extraordinarily seductive.

Spinning Freud's phylogenetic fantasy further, he then of course sketches, in the form of an enlightened utopia, psychoanalysis' task of secularization:

I clearly understand the anxiety phase, the hysteria and obsession phase—also, by the way, presumed in the case of the child. What is quite new and surprising is the parallel drawn between the struggle against the father and the later types of neurosis. The religious phase of mankind (which still persists), with the exaggerated sense of sin, seems to be the last offshoot of melancholia. Psychoanalysis signifies mankind's convalescence, the emancipation from religion, from (unjustified) authority and from the exaggerated rebellion against it; thus, the beginning of the scientific (objective) phase.

In conclusion, Ferenczi formulates an objection,[9] as well as several additions:

Only the analogy between dementia praecox and the castration phase is not clear to me. The castrated ones cannot have reproduced and fixated their condition phylogenetically; therefore you must mean the fixation of castration *anxiety*. To be sure, the loss of the mother could at first have resulted in complete helplessness and regression to narcissism on the part of the expelled sons. But the question is,

7. As Freud indicates in the draft (p. 11 and p. 16), this phrase relates to Ferenczi's paper "Stages in the Development of the Sense of Reality" (1913). It also relates to the "bioanalytic" studies on a theory of coitus, which were occupying Ferenczi at the time and about which he occasionally reported to Freud in his letters of this period, but which were not published until 1924 in *Thalassa: A Theory of Genitality*. See "The Work Context," below.

8. Here the transcription reads *mit* (with).

9. It is this objection that Freud designates as "fortunately . . . anticipated" in his brief letter on the back of the last page of the manuscript of the draft (above, pp. xvi–xvii).

how can this phase have been phylogenetically fixated? The fixation of homosexuality is equally enigmatic, unless one assumes that individual homosexuals remained bisexual and were able to reproduce. It would be the case that each of these phases brought about individual "criminals" who, unhindered by the prevailing current of the time, copulated normally with the woman (mother). (Oedipus, rape of the Sabine women.)[10]

Freud thanks Ferenczi briefly on July 27, saying, "Your long-awaited comments about the phylogenetic series were very welcome and put the matter in a further state of flux." On the following day he sends Ferenczi the draft. And on July 31 he concludes: "You will find the answer to your criticism of the phylogenetic series in the enclosed 'draft.' " Ferenczi evidently responds with a long, original letter, which he asks Freud to return to him inasmuch as it probably contained thoughts he wanted to pursue in his own studies. On August 9 Freud complies with this request: "I am reluctantly returning to you this significant letter, in which I recognize the matrix of several important endeavors."[11] It closes with the laconic statement, "The twelve papers are, so to speak, finished."

Thereafter the correspondence becomes increasingly silent with regard to the metapsychological writings. When Freud suggests on October 31 that Ferenczi "stick" his planned bioanalytic essays "into the next volume of the yearbook," in other words fill it with these texts so that it could be published, he says not a word about his own unpublished papers. On December 6 he reports on a "great diplomatic success," namely that he has persuaded his publisher, Hugo Heller, "to take both of my books and, in exchange, to keep the journal going." The two books were the *Introductory Lectures on Psycho-Analysis* (1916–17 [1915–17]), which Freud had begun in the second half of 1915, and the metapsychology. With respect to the latter he adds, of course, that Heller "wanted to bring it out a while later."

The discussion between the friends about the metapsychology probably continued verbally, because on March 24 of the following year Freud asked Ferenczi, to whom he had evidently given the manuscripts of the unpublished papers for review, to return them during a visit to Vienna. "I

10. Freud tried to invalidate these reservations, with a logic that occasionally sounds somewhat nitpicking, in a supplement to his draft, namely (as he indicates in the accompanying letter) pp. 21–23 of the manuscript, which correspond to pp. 19–20 of the edited version—from "Now it is time . . . " to the end of the text.

11. Apparently Ferenczi later threw the letter away. In any case it is not in the transcribed Freud-Ferenczi correspondence.

am thinking of abandoning the paper about the Cs. and replacing it with a more appropriate one, for example, 'The Three Viewpoints of MΨ' [Metapsychology]." As a result, not only did the publisher hesitate, but Freud himself was dissatisfied. In a gloomy mood—sometimes "I have to struggle for a long time until I regain my mental equilibrium"—and filled with thoughts of death, he reported to Ferenczi more than a year later, on November 20, 1917: "In a kind of urge to set my house in order I have sent two of the essays on metapsychology (Mourning and Melancholia, A Metapsychological Supplement to the Theory of Dreams) to Sachs for the last issue of the journal. (The rest may be kept quiet.)"

Nothing in Freud's attitude toward "the rest" changed in the ensuing period. When during the last months of the war, on March 17, 1918, he informed Ferenczi about his latest plans for publication, the metapsychology remained unnamed. Indeed, when Lou Andreas-Salomé stubbornly asked him once again on March 18, 1919, he explained, at first glance surprisingly:[12] "What has happened to my *Metapsychology?* In the first place, it remains unwritten" (1966a [1912–36], p. 95). That is, after the war he no longer regarded what had been set forth in the seven unpublished papers as a successful synthesis of his theoretical conceptions, and he gave up the plan to publish the book.

One may speculate about the reasons for this change of heart. Probably of least significance was the fact that portions of the texts had not been finally edited and coordinated and thus did not meet the high formal standards of Freud, the writer. This deficiency would have been easy to eliminate, had not other more weighty reasons discouraged publication.

Although in all his creative phases Freud was a great, bold systematizer and synthesizer, he apparently placed little value on this trait of his intellectual temperament and even disavowed it at times. He preferred to emphasize the empirical, the inductive aspect of his approach. While he was still writing the metapsychological papers, he mentioned in a letter of June 7, 1915, to James J. Putnam "my own way of restricting myself to what lies nearest, is most tangible, and yet is actually petty . . . I am somewhat frightened by uncertainty. I am timid rather than courageous and gladly sacrifice much for the feeling that I am on solid ground" (1971a [1906–

12. Because on May 25, 1916, he had informed her: "My book consisting of twelve essays of this kind cannot be published before the end of the war. And who knows how long after that ardently longed-for date?"

16]), pp. 187–188). On several occasions Freud explained to Lou Andreas-Salomé how he worked: "step by step," according to a letter of July 13, 1917, "without the inner need for completion, continually under the pressure of the problem immediately on hand, and taking infinite pains not to be diverted from the path." In the cited letter of April 2, 1919, in which Freud pointblank declares that the metapsychology "remains unwritten," he continues, as if in justification, "The systematic working through of material is not possible for me; the fragmentary nature of my experiences and the sporadic character of my insights do not permit it."

Of the seven unpublished and later lost metapsychological papers, the twelfth, judging by the draft, may have been the one that in its second part was furthest from clinical experience.[13] From the beginning Freud recognized and cited the speculative character of his phylogenetic reflections, and not only in the letters to Ferenczi. It is equally emphasized in the draft, which the fair copy followed "sentence for sentence," that the reader "should allow himself some hypothetical link" in the argumentation and that it is a matter of "scientific fantasies."

In the letter of July 12, 1915, transcribed above in its entirety, Freud sketches for Ferenczi for the first time the content of his overview of the transference neuroses and says at the outset that he is dealing with fantasies that trouble him. We may elaborate: they troubled him, the person who had laboriously "learned to restrain speculative tendencies" (1914d, p. 22), precisely *because* these were fantasies. In another connection, but still as if he wanted indirectly to pull himself together after writing the draft, he declares in a letter to Ferenczi sent only three days after the draft, "I maintain that one should not make theories—they must fall into one's house as uninvited guests while one is occupied with the investigation of details." A few months earlier, on April 8, in the middle of the work on his metapsychological writings, Freud had concisely and memorably described to Ferenczi the "mechanism" of scientific creativity as the "succession of daringly playful fantasy and relentlessly realistic criticism." We can assume that the daringly, all too daringly, playful fantasy in the second part of the twelfth metapsychological paper did not stand up to the subsequent relentlessly realistic criticism.

13. At least, this position can be maintained with regard to the four other texts, whose themes Freud mentioned in his letters: consciousness, anxiety, conversion hysteria, obsessional neurosis. Strachey (1957a, p. 106) speculates that the two other papers had to do with sublimation and projection (or paranoia), thus likewise with clinical problems.

But what caused Freud in the end to reject the other, presumably far less speculative, texts as well? Only after the war would he finally have been able to publish his book on the preliminaries to a metapsychology. By then, however, he was already occupied with quite different theoretical trains of thought, which would have forced a complete revision of these now outdated chapters. Since March 1919 he had been working on a first draft of *Beyond the Pleasure Principle* (1920g). This book introduced the new instinct-dualism—life and death instincts, whereas the metapsychological papers still start from the earlier classification—sexual instincts and ego-instincts. Against the background of his growing insight into the unconscious functioning of defense mechanisms and the resulting crystallization of structural theory and ego psychology, it comes as no surprise that Freud was particularly dissatisfied with the chapter on consciousness. He must have been similarly uncomfortable with the anxiety paper, because it presumably was still broadly based on his earlier, toxicological theory of anxiety. This is supported in the remarks about anxiety in the draft overview.[14]

The Work Context

In giving the first indications about his work on the metapsychological papers in the letter of November 25, 1914, Freud informed Ferenczi that he was moving "on paths that have been trodden for a long time." Without intending here to reconstruct the various developmental stages of Freudian metapsychology,[15] I remind the reader that the word surfaces for the first time in Freud's letters to Wilhelm Fliess, specifically in the letter of February 13, 1896. More detailed commentary follows in the letter of March 10, 1898, where, in connection with a remark about the dream book (1900a), Freud says: "It seems to me that the theory of wish fulfillment has brought only the psychological solution and not the biological—or, rather, metapsychical—one. (I am going to ask you seriously, by the way, whether I may use the term metapsychology for my psychology that leads behind consciousness.)" (1985, pp. 301–302). In the *Psycho-*

14. "The Unconscious" (1915e), to be sure, contains one hint (p. 183) that the development of small quantities of anxiety can be used as a signal.

15. See for instance Nagera (1970, pp. 19–46).

pathology of Everyday Life (1901b, pp. 258–259) Freud had acknowledged that in the choice of the name he had indeed intended a parallel to metaphysics:

> I believe that a large part of the mythological view of the world, which extends a long way into the most modern religions, *is nothing but psychology projected into the external world.* The obscure recognition (the endopsychic perception, as it were) of psychical factors and relations in the unconscious is mirrored . . . in the construction of a *supernatural reality,* which is destined to be changed back once more by science into the *psychology of the unconscious.* One could venture to explain in this way the myths of paradise and the fall of man, of God, of good and evil, of immortality, and so on, and to transform *metaphysics* into *metapsychology.*

It was not until 1915, in the central metapsychological paper on "The Unconscious" (1915e) that Freud defined metapsychology precisely, in a way that has maintained its validity for psychoanalysis: "I propose that when we have succeeded in describing a psychical process in its dynamic, topographical, and economic aspects, we should speak of it as a *metapsychological* presentation" (p. 181). Yet certainly not all works in which Freud described psychical processes in this way should be termed metapsychological. It is customary today to count as Freud's major metapsychological works only those writings in which he unfolds his theoretical thoughts explicitly, exclusively, and in detail at the highest level of abstraction—as the "consummation of psycho-analytic research" (ibid.). These writings are the "Project for a Scientific Psychology" (1950a [1895]), which dates from the preanalytic period; the seventh chapter of *The Interpretation of Dreams;* the "Formulations on the Two Principles of Mental Functioning" (1911b); "On Narcissism: An Introduction" (1914c); the five published metapsychological papers of 1915; *Beyond the Pleasure Principle* (1920g); and *The Ego and the Id* (1923b).[16]

The question of how the twelfth metapsychological paper might have been woven into the fabric of the total work and whether, when Freud finally rejected it, threads were left hanging forever or were taken up again in other, later works, cannot be answered fully so soon after the reemergence of the draft. What follows are no more than initial speculations on some of the themes.

16. One can of course extend the concept—as was done, for instance, by the editors of the *Studienausgabe,* who also count other works of Freud collected in vol. 3 of that edition as metapsychology.

The structure of the text shows a striking two-part division. It lends itself to proceeding in two steps, that is, examining this question in first the one, then the other part. The first part encompasses a systematic comparison of the six factors that operate in the three transference neuroses. Proceeding inductively, all statements build on "careful and arduous observation" and are strictly limited to the ontogenetic level. Freud believed he had to ascribe "boredom" to these sections, perhaps an echo of his own frame of mind when he formulated them. Beginning with the sixth factor, on page 10, the involvement of the inherited disposition in the etiology of the neuroses, it is as if the moorings are broken. The second part—the adventure of the phylogenetic reconstruction—follows and, breaking the bounds of the draft's title, forces inclusion of the "narcissistic neuroses." Here Freud permits himself, at least for the moment of writing (as he himself clearly admitted), to let "criticism retreat in the face of fantasy" and to bring forth deductively derived "unconfirmed things."

That he was treading on rather familiar ground in the first part is shown not least by the large number of omitted words and abbreviations; the first part has a much more pronounced shorthand character than the second, which is almost completely written out.[17] As Freud says at the beginning of the draft, it is a matter of summarizing and comparing after the preliminary "detailed investigation." As mentioned, in the six other lost metapsychological papers anxiety hysteria, conversion hysteria, and obsessional neurosis (among other subjects) were studied, so that in the overview Freud could confine himself to reminding the reader, through brief characterizations, of the individual factors.

Following Freud's train of thought presents no great difficulty, even without knowledge of the lost texts. Repression, anticathexis, substitutive- and symptom-formation, sexual function, regression, fixation and disposition—the six factors are like the warp in the fabric of the total work, never given up, elaborated upon if need be, and varied in the course of decisive conceptual innovations.[18] It would go beyond the framework

17. This is, of course, much more apparent in the manuscript (see the facsimile and the transcription, which is totally faithful to it) than in the edited version, where abbreviations have been written out in the interest of readability. In the tidied-up fair copy, it is possible that the proportions were different: the first part, which corresponds to the title of the paper, might have taken up more space than the second.

18. To give only one example, the draft is still concerned with the broader concept of repression in the general sense of defense. Only later (1926d [1925]) did Freud use the term

of the present considerations to pursue these changes (even with respect to only one of the six factors) in those of Freud's works that originated at about this time—such as the *Introductory Lectures on Psychoanalysis* (1916–17 [1915–17]), where there are constructions similar to those in the draft, including the choice of words. It would also go beyond our present considerations to explore them in his later writings, for instance, in *Inhibitions, Symptoms and Anxiety* (1926d). In that work, in a manner very similar to that of the first part of the overview, Freud again and again compares the three transference neuroses in relation to the individual factors.[19]

Whoever consults the five published metapsychological papers of 1915 will be able to visualize in particular the specific context of Freudian theory formation in which the twelfth paper would have belonged. Moreover, in "Repression" (1915d) and "The Unconscious" (1915e) five of the six factors of the overview are already dealt with in more or less detail, in one form or another. At the end of "Repression" there is even a first *comparative* investigation of the process of repression in the three transference neuroses.[20] Here, as later in the overview, the questions of success or failure, the relation of symptom- and substitutive-formation, the connection with the instinctual vicissitudes of regression are also taken into consideration. Indeed, the last paragraph of "Repression" reads like a preview of some of the seven lost papers, in particular the comparative first part of the twelfth:

The extraordinary intricacy of all the factors to be taken into consideration leaves only one way of presenting them open to us. We must select first one and then another point of view, and follow it up through the material as long as the application of it seems to yield results. Each separate treatment of the subject will

---

consistently in the limited sense of the defense mechanism specific to hysteria. In "Repression" (1915d, pp. 153–154), certainly, there is already a hint of this differentiation.

19. Examples occur in one of the addenda about anticathexis (pp. 157–160) and in the fifth chapter concerning symptom-formation. As in the draft, we find reference to a temporal ranking of the appearance of the three disorders in childhood, as well as a phylogenetic discussion in the context of the diphasic nature of human sexual life. In fact, it seems as though Freud, years later, in *Inhibitions, Symptoms and Anxiety* consciously resumed and worked out many trains of thought from the first part of his rejected twelfth metapsychological paper, using them as material enriched by the concepts of the structural theory that had been added in the meantime, to unfold his second theory of anxiety. (Such a resumption of earlier material would provide a reasonable explanation for the unevenness of this book, justifiably criticized by Strachey, 1959, p. 78.)

20. See also a similar comparative attempt at the end of the fourth section, Topography and Dynamics of Repression, in "The Unconscious" (1915e, pp. 180–185).

be incomplete in itself, and there cannot fail to be obscurities where it touches upon material that has not yet been treated; but we may hope that a final synthesis will lead to a proper understanding. (1915d, pp. 157–158)

Although we lack the fair copy of the "final synthesis" in the form of the first part of the overview of the transference neuroses, we can presume with some certainty on the basis of the draft and the contents of the five published metapsychology texts of 1915 that no fundamentally new theoretical ideas have perished with the loss of the seven pieces.[21]

Of the six factors the *one* that is only briefly mentioned in the published metapsychological papers of 1915 is also named last in the first part of the draft: disposition, "the most decisive factor, the one that mediates the decision concerning [the] choice of neurosis." In "Instincts and Their Vicissitudes" (1915c, p. 120) Freud mentions in passing that muscular movements which turn out to be purposeful in mastering external stimuli become "a hereditary disposition"; but "instinctual stimuli, which originate from within the organism, cannot be dealt with by this mechanism . . . There is naturally nothing to prevent our supposing that the instincts themselves are, at least in part, precipitates of the effects of external stimulation, which in the course of phylogenesis have brought about modifications in the living substance." A few pages later (p. 131) is a sentence about instinctual life "in primaeval times" in relation to what Freud conceived of as "archaic inheritance." "Mourning and Melancholia" (1917e [1915]) tells us that "the disposition to fall ill of melancholia" can be seen in the "predominance of the narcissistic type of object-choice" (p. 250); this is cited as a conclusion required "[by] theory"—which, to be sure, lacks

21. Of particular interest in the section on regression are a few brief remarks about ego regression in conversion hysteria, specifically with regard to the more recent discussion of hysteria (for example, the ideas presented in the hysteria panel of the Twenty-eighth Congress of the International Psychoanalytical Association in Paris in 1973, or Masud R. Khan's paper of 1974). Some of these authors have specifically addressed Freud's early concept of hysteria. When Freud speaks in his draft of the return to a psychical level "without separation of Pcs. and Ucs., thus without speech and censorship" he means functional modalities of the ego from the preverbal time of the mother-child dyad. He of course explains this regression differently than do the above-mentioned authors—namely, drive-dynamically, as in the service of the return of the repressed. Khan, for instance, places the causation of hysterical illness in this phase of the earliest development of the ego. He sees it in the mother's failure to recognize and satisfy the earliest ego needs of the child. He also sees it in the child's attempt, by means of precocious sexualization, to master the resulting psychical or psychophysical condition of deprivation through an intensification of the experiences of the body ego instead of the unfolding of mental ego functions.

empirical confirmation. In the next paragraph there is casual mention of the "disposition to obsessional neurosis,"[22] both times in the ontogenetic sense. A few lines later the conflict due to ambivalence is confirmed as arising "sometimes . . . more from real experiences, sometimes more from constitutional factors" (p. 251), where "constitutional," or "constitutive"[23] (pp. 256–257), means solely that it is a matter of a regularly present tendency to conflict in the particular individual. "The Unconscious" (1915e, p. 195), says, however: "The content of the *Ucs.* may be compared with an aboriginal population of the mind. If inherited mental formations exist in the human being—something analogous to instinct in animals—these constitute the nucleus of the *Ucs.*" This is the only prominent reference in the five published metapsychological papers of 1915 to the phylogenetic dimension in depth that Freud prepared to penetrate in the second part of his twelfth paper.

For the second, radically different part of the draft, with its truly breathtaking "widening of the horizon," Freud sets the stage, as it were, in the second and third paragraphs of section (f) for a gripping phylogenetic playlet in two acts and six scenes, set in the early period of the history of our race. In the first act, after a paradisiacal prehistory, rages the "struggle with the exigencies of the Ice Age," which leads to the "patriarchal stage of civilization." Its three scenes depict the events and phases of the human condition, which precipitated out in the hereditary disposition to the three transference neuroses (anxiety hysteria, conversion hysteria, obsessional neurosis). The dramatic origin of the fixations on which the three narcissistic neuroses (dementia praecox, paranoia, melancholia-mania) are phylogenetically based is the theme of the three subsequent scenes of the second act. It is set in the time after the end of the Ice Age, in the phase of the oppression of the primal father, who had become tyrannical; and it portrays the development of the social stage of civilization, which succeeds the patriarchal stage.

22. This is an echo of the title of Freud's paper of the same name (1913i), which appeared two years earlier. As the subtitle says, it represents a "contribution to the problem of the choice of neurosis," which had occupied Freud since the 1890s and which from the beginning he had viewed from the perspective of biological evolution. There are many other cross-connections to "The Disposition to Obsessional Neurosis": for example, there (pp. 318 ff.) one also finds factors relative to the sequential appearance of the various psychoneurotic disorders in the life cycle.

23. ⟨In these passages Freud uses two different German terms, *konstitutiv* and *konstitutionell.* Strachey translates both as "constitutional."⟩

In contrast to the first part of the draft, Freud in the second makes reference to the work context. He mentions three of his writings.

He cites first the "Formulations on the Two Principles of Mental Functioning" (1911b), specifically in connection with the statement that a different development is to be ascribed to the sexual strivings of man than to the ego strivings. In the pertinent passages the discussion is, in fact (just as in the draft), about disposition and choice of neurosis, but again in the ontogenetic sense.

Freud's naming of *Totem and Taboo* (1912–13)—his first great contribution to the theory of civilization—is directly illuminating for the work context. This reference to the literature is found, not coincidentally, at the point in the draft where he talks about the sons "to whom the jealous primal father does not allow full scope." As is well known, *Totem and Taboo* discusses for the first time the "great event with which civilization began and which, since it occurred, has not allowed mankind a moment's rest" (p. 145); it addresses the "primaeval tragedy" (p. 156), which Freud unfolds in the draft. There in the fourth essay he establishes the connection between the animal phobias of children and the original motives of totemism, then links up with Darwin's theses (1871) about the primal condition of society, about early man's living in small hordes. He makes these connections in order to develop, finally, following James Jasper Atkinson (1903),[24] his vehemently disputed "hypothesis, which has such a monstrous air, of the tyrannical father being overwhelmed and killed by a combination of his exiled sons" (p. 142n). Freud was destined to adhere to this hypothesis as a basic statement on human aggression, as it were, inviolably for the rest of his life.[25] In *Totem and Taboo,* to be sure, he does in several places still bring methodological reservations to the fore and concedes that this hypothesis could "seem fantastic" (p. 141); he expressly mentions the "uncertainties of my premises" (p. 157), even where he concerns himself with the hereditary passing on of the guilt feeling that ensues from the murderous act.

24. See esp. chaps. 2 and 3, where "parricidal crime" (p. 225) is discussed. See also note 48 below.

25. See, for example, 1921c, pp. 122–128, 135–137; 1930a [1929], pp. 100, 131–132; 1939a [1934–38], pp. 130–132. At the last location (p. 131) is a late commentary of Freud's on his refusal to modify the hypotheses developed in *Totem and Taboo* in light of more recent results of cultural-anthropological research. For a comprehensive presentation of the critical perspectives on these hypotheses within and without cultural anthropology, from the publication of the book to the present, see Wallace (1983), esp. chaps. 4 and 5.

I have supposed that the sense of guilt for an action has persisted for many thousands of years and has remained operative in generations which can have had no knowledge of that action. I have supposed that an emotional process, such as might have developed in generations of sons who were ill-treated by their father, has extended to new generations which were exempt from such treatment for the very reason that their father had been eliminated . . . This gives rise to two . . . questions: How much can we attribute to psychical continuity in the sequence of generations? and what are the ways and means employed by one generation in order to hand on its mental states to the next one? I shall not pretend that these problems are sufficiently explained or that direct communication and tradition—which are the first things that occur to one—are enough to account for the process . . . A part of the problem seems to be met by the inheritance of psychical dispositions which, however, need to be given some sort of impetus in the life of the individual before they can be roused into actual operation. (pp. 157–158)

Against the background of these formulations the twelfth metapsychological paper reads like a variation on the great theme struck in *Totem and Taboo*.

The third of his own works mentioned by Freud is the *Three Essays on the Theory of Sexuality* (1905d). He refers to the essays laconically, in connection with the statement: "[As for] the development of human sexual life, we believe we have learned to understand it in broad outline." In a letter to Ferenczi of December 2, 1914, he had flatly referred to the newly begun work on the metapsychological writings as a "continuation of the problems where I left off with them in the sexual theory." The revolutionary work may in the final analysis have been so active in Freud's mind while he was writing the draft, not least because he was at about the same time preparing the third, thoroughly revised edition of the *Three Essays*. From the preface to the new edition of 1915:

Throughout . . . preference is given to the accidental factors, while disposition is left in the background, and more weight is attached to ontogenesis than to phylogenesis. For it is the accidental factors that play the principal part in analysis: they are almost entirely subject to its influence. The dispositional ones only come to light after them, as something stirred into activity by experience . . . The relation between ontogenesis and phylogenesis is a similar one. Ontogenesis may be regarded as a recapitulation of phylogenesis . . . But disposition is ultimately the precipitate of earlier experience of the species to which the more recent experience of the individual, as the sum of the accidental factors, is super-added. (p. 131)[26]

26. Freud had already discussed something similar in a letter of October 1, 1911, to Else Voigtländer (1960a, pp. 283–285).

The phylogenetic considerations introduced in connection with the metapsychological papers have left conspicuous traces, not only in the preface to the new edition of the *Three Essays,* but also in numerous additions to the text—for example, in the concluding passage (pp. 239–240).

The *Three Essays* surface again and again too in the letters Freud exchanged with Ferenczi during the war years, and not only in connection with the work on the revisions for the third edition. Ferenczi, stationed since the fall of 1914 in the small garrison town of Pápa, translated the book into Hungarian, which stimulated him to enthusiastic rereading and unleashed a storm of thoughts in the direction of biology. Close inspection shows that in the second part of the draft Freud not only makes reference to his own work context, he refers to still another work context by twice emphasizing Ferenczi's investigation of the "Stages in the Development of the Sense of Reality" (1913). Ferenczi, to be sure, basically argues on the ontogenetic plane, but still assumes a "transference of the memory traces of the race's history on to the individual" (pp. 219–220) and at the end ventures a "scientific prophecy" to the effect that

> it was the geological changes in the surface of the earth, with their catastrophic consequences for primitive man, that compelled repression of favourite habits and thus "development." Such catastrophes may have been the sites of repression in the history of racial development, and the temporal localization and intensity of such catastrophes may have decided the character and the neuroses of the race. (p. 237)

These formulations make it understandable why Freud, in the above-quoted letter to Ferenczi of July 12, 1915, added to the end of the first sketch of his phylogenetic fantasy the sentence, "Your priority in all this is evident."

The intensity and character of the two friends' collaboration during the period in which the twelfth metapsychological paper originated have already been pointed out. Their cooperation encompassed more than just the overview, however. That Freud ultimately abandoned the project is in no small measure bound up with the vicissitudes of their discussion about basic questions of biology—or, as Ferenczi called it, "metabiology." Its reconstruction from the unpublished correspondence will, moreover, facilitate consideration of the historicoscientific context, in which the second section of the draft belongs, as among those components of Freud's metapsychology that refer to evolutionary biology.

While Freud was still working on the first metapsychological papers, Ferenczi had complained to him on February 2, 1915: "I have got carried away with *biological* problems and can't find my way back to psychology! . . . It is interesting to observe the great pattern that expresses itself in the reaction of both of us to the idleness forced upon us by the war. One now understands the speculative biologists and philosophers, who—always far removed from reality—would like to build the entire world edifice upon the few facts known to them." Stimulated by his translation of the *Three Essays,* Ferenczi immersed himself in theoretical considerations, about which he informed Freud on March 18 "that it has to do with a new theory of coitus, which seems to me appropriate for unifying *all* (almost all) of the points of your theory of sexuality. When I have put the notes, which are now in disarray, into halfway-decent order, I will come once more to Vienna to present the matter to you."

Freud evidently felt stimulated by this exchange of views to the extent that he wrote to Ferenczi on July 20, 1915, a few days after sending him the sketch in his letter (p. 79 above): "I was considering alluding only briefly to the phylogenetic series with reference to your work and with fitting commendation of your fruitful and original idea about the influence of the geological vicissitudes. Now, however, you have given me the desire for a more extensive presentation, which I will attempt and will show you before I make a decision about publication." In the meantime Ferenczi developed his "plan for a series of essays," formally modeled on Freud's metapsychology project, "entitled *Bioanalytic Essays;* it could be about fifteen to twenty papers, which could ultimately fill a book. The first paper will be generally 'On the Justification of Psychoanalytic Points of View in the Biological Sphere of Knowledge' and will confirm the naturalness of and the necessity for the metapsychological and metabiological way of looking at things" (letter of October 26, 1915).

Like Freud's book project, Ferenczi's metabiology plan soon came to a standstill. The phylogenetic thoughts, however, continued to be pursued on the side. Thus, Freud writes on January 6, 1916: "Don't we now know two conditions for artistic endowment? First, the wealth of phylogenetically transferred material, as with the neurotic; second, a good remnant of the old technique of modifying oneself instead of the outside world (see Lamarck, etc.)." So here, finally, appears the name of the natural scientist whose concepts, especially in their psycho-Lamarckian extensions, have—indirectly, of course—helped mold the phylogenetic fantasy.

From this point on, Lamarck is mentioned more frequently for a while in the correspondence; during the infrequent meetings of the two friends the idea took shape to write something jointly about Lamarckism and psychoanalysis.[27] At the end of the year, on December 22, 1916, a letter of Freud's states that he ordered "the Lamarck" in the university library. "I cannot stay completely idle, and our project, 'L and PsA,' suddenly came to mind as hopeful and rich in content." A few days later, on December 28, Ferenczi confirmed the "joint plan of work." On the first day of 1917 Freud sent a "sketch of the Lamarck-work," a paper apparently not preserved, and reported that he had begun reading the *Zoological Philosophy* (1963 [1809]), the work that stands at the beginning of the development of a scientific theory of descent. In a rapid succession of letters suggestions were then exchanged about the procedure for obtaining the literature as well as for dividing up the work, and notes and suggestions for precise wording were sent back and forth.

But the initial élan soon began to fade. On the one hand, because of the war, there were difficulties in getting the literature. On the other hand, what was obtained and read seems to have led to a rude awakening. Freud concedes on January 28, 1917: "My impression is that we are coming completely into line with the psycho-Lamarckists, such as Pauly, and will have little to say that is completely new. Still, PsA will then have left its calling card with biology." Ultimately the external emergency situation, which was reaching crisis level, may also have had an inhibiting effect: in a letter of the following March 2 Freud strives to alleviate Ferenczi's self-reproaches by assuring him that "you need not worry about neglecting our work on Lamarck. I have not progressed either; in the weeks of cold and darkness I stopped working in the evening—and have not got back to it since then." And on May 29 he writes, "I am not at all disposed to doing the work on Lamarck in the summer and would prefer to relinquish the whole thing to you."[28]

Basically, this is what transpired. At the end of the year, on December 27, Freud addresses the subject in similar fashion: "I cannot make up my mind about getting back to Lamarck. Perhaps our problem with him is

27. See Jones (1955, pp. 194–195).

28. That Freud considered Ferenczi the most competent biologist among his collaborators he had already assured him on April 29, 1916, in another context: "I maintain that this is your real field, in which you will be without peer."

like that of the two noble Poles and their bill: 'because neither one could bear to have the other one pay for him, neither one paid.' "[29] On May 18, 1918, Ferenczi applied pressure for the last time: "It would be good if the *work on Lamarck* took recognizable shape this summer." But Freud waved him off. Shortly before the end of the war, on October 16, he explained: "Not disposed to work . . . too much interested in the end of the world drama."

Subsequently the literary interests of the two went their separate ways. In the spring of 1919 Freud reported on new labors, on "A Child Is Being Beaten" (1919e), and, with growing excitement, on *Beyond the Pleasure Principle* (1920g). From a letter of Ferenczi dated March 18, 1919, we may infer that some of his own plans were also coming to fruition, "for instance, the one about the final realization of the paleobiological speculations." But Ferenczi still required several years before he could make a decision about publishing his *Thalassa: A Theory of Genitality* (1968 [1924]);[30] and then not without first having inquired of Freud in a letter of July 25, 1923, "Will you permit me . . . (in the biological part) to come back to the assumptions about Lamarckism that were jointly constructed in Pápa and elsewhere?" At several points in the published version of *Thalassa* we are able to recognize offshoots of this—where, for instance, Ferenczi conceives of symbols as "historically significant traces of 'repressed' biological situations" (p. 87); or where he attempts, in the sense of a "depth biology" (p. 84), to "insinuate a novel theory of evolution and development in which we simply transferred to the biological sphere psychoanalytic findings and assumptions regarding developmental pro-

29. ⟨This quotation is from a satirical poem by Heinrich Heine entitled *Zwei Ritter* (Two knights).⟩ The demise of the Lamarck project may have been hastened by the fact that Ferenczi vainly attempted during these years to resume his prematurely terminated analysis with Freud, a thesis that cannot be examined here in more detail.

30. Of course, there are a wealth of implicit and explicit cross-references between *Beyond the Pleasure Principle* and *Thalassa*. It was clear in Freud's mind that the speculative thought principle of the discussions with Ferenczi during the war years continued to have an effect in *Beyond the Pleasure Principle* (esp. pp. 58–61; see also Paniagua, 1982). Lamarckian-biogenetic perspectives continue too in *The Ego and the Id* (1923b, sec. 3, in connection with considerations about the origin of the super-ego); Freud emphasizes that he is here pursuing the trains of thought begun in *Beyond the Pleasure Principle,* but without "fresh borrowings from biology"; for that reason, in his view, this paper is closer to psychoanalysis than the other and is "more in the nature of a synthesis than of a speculation" (p. 12). Moreover, there is a later reference (p. 35) to the significance of the Ice Age for the development of civilization. For continuation of the Freud-Ferenczian phylogenetic-biogenetic ideas some years later see Balint (1930).

cesses in the psychological realm" (p. 88); or, finally, where he explicitly claims to

> have no reason for disbelieving that such wishful strivings operate also outside the psychic and therefore in the biological unconscious; indeed, we are inclined to feel and may boast of being in accord with Freud therein, that the adjuvant rôle played by the wish as a factor in evolution makes the Lamarckian theory of adaptation for the first time intelligible. (pp. 90–91)

Thalassa: A Theory of Genitality is thus both the legacy of the abandoned Lamarck project and, in a certain sense, also of the rejected "Phylogenetic Fantasy." It shares with the latter the adventurous beauty of the speculative flight of fancy, the brilliant reconstruction of a primeval drama about human phylogenesis, the peculiar mélange of scientific raw material and literary treatment.[31] Freud's former fascination with the joint metapsychological-metabiological intellectual excursions of the war years still resounds in 1933 in the otherwise ambivalent obituary to Ferenczi. There, with regard to the "summit of achievement" of *Thalassa,* he says—as if it were simultaneously the obituary notice of his own phylogenetic fantasy—"perhaps the boldest application of psycho-analysis that was ever attempted . . . one finds oneself the richer for hints that promise a deep insight into wide fields of biology. It is a vain task to attempt already today to distinguish what can be accepted as an authentic discovery from what seeks, in the fashion of a scientific phantasy, to guess at future knowledge" (1933c, p. 228).[32]

Yet it would be wrong to believe that Freud had, so to speak, "relinquished" the whole thought complex of his unpublished phylogenetic fantasy to Ferenczi. Just as many themes do not emerge for the first time in the second part of the draft, neither do they appear there for the last

31. This sort of mélange is a form of presentation that was not unusual for the time. It also characterizes, for example, in even more extreme form, the work by Wittels (1912), cited by Freud in the draft and designated flatly in its subtitle as "primeval fiction."

32. Reading this extraordinary book today, one can still imagine future biologists' rediscovering *Thalassa* as an artistic and at the same time brilliantly abstruse anticipation of revolutionary biological concepts. Although these concepts are only now beginning to be developed, someday when they are properly elaborated, they may help to achieve a completely new theoretical level of understanding of the life processes; they will probably make the Lamarckian-Darwinian discussion seem antiquated and a false formulation of the question. If so, this would mean that Freud and Ferenczi, with their metapsychological-metabiological speculations, were even farther ahead of the biology of their time than, with psychoanalysis in a narrower sense, they were ahead of the psychology of their day.

time. Only one—today certainly a sore point in the reading—should be mentioned briefly: the differences between the sexes. To be sure, Freud later on no longer let himself be carried away by the exaggerated claim that the beginnings of mastery over nature, law, investigation, thinking, even speech, were predominantly the cultural achievements of males. Nevertheless, some of his later expositions about the gender-specific differences in the structure of the super-ego[33] read like more or less moderated variations on the trains of thought sketched out in the draft. Furthermore, his later writings on the subject are characterized by the striking preponderance of statements on the development of the male. Indeed, the formulation the "vicissitudes of women in these primeval times are especially obscure to us" even reminds us in the choice of words of the "*dark continent*" (1926e, p. 212)—an expression Freud used to describe the view of modern female sexuality that he probably held for the rest of his life. But not merely individual themes can be identified in earlier and later texts of Freud; the basic biogenetic-Lamarckian concepts, including the idea of the inheritability of archaic layers of the world of symbols, run like a warp through the fabric of his total work.

The Historicoscientific Context

Freud continued to work on this warp[34] in the *Introductory Lectures on Psycho-Analysis* (1916–17 [1915–17]), which originated almost simultaneously. This continuity is illustrated in the reference to the archaic characteristics of dreams, where he explains succinctly: "It seems to me, for instance, that symbolic connections, which the individual has never acquired by learning, may justly claim to be regarded as a phylogenetic heritage" (vol. 15, p. 199). In another example he follows the paths of symptom-formation and designates primal fantasies as phylogenetic endowment: "The individual reaches beyond his own experience into primaeval experience" (vol. 16, p. 371).[35] In the final analysis it sounds like

33. See, for example, 1923b, p. 37; 1925j, pp. 257–258; 1933a, p. 134.

34. It can be traced back to the beginning of Freud's work. See, for instance, Draft B of February 8, 1893, from the communications to Wilhelm Fliess (1985, pp. 39–44).

35. In *Totem and Taboo* (p. 31) Freud had expressed himself much more cautiously: "[These prohibitions] must . . . have persisted from generation to generation, perhaps merely as a result of tradition transmitted through parental and social authority. Possibly, however, in later genera-

a recollection of the rejected phylogenetic fantasy, when he summarizes: "I have repeatedly been led to suspect that the psychology of the neuroses has stored up in it more of the antiquities of human development than any other source" (ibid.). Freud expressed similar thoughts in a subsequent postscript to the case history of the Wolf-Man (1918b [1914], p. 97) and in *The Ego and the Id* (1923b, pp. 37–38).

In spite of all the criticism leveled against Lamarckian explanations in the meantime, Freud held fast to them to the end. As in the late *Outline of Psycho-Analysis* (1940a [1938], pp. 167, 207), he still insisted in his book on Moses (1939a [1934–38]) that "the archaic heritage of human beings comprises not only dispositions but also subject-matter—memory-traces of the experience of earlier generations" (p. 99). Not that this criticism had escaped him:[36]

> On further reflection I must admit that I have behaved for a long time as though the inheritance of memory-traces of the experience of our ancestors, independently of direct communication and of the influence of education by the setting of an example, were established beyond question . . . My position, no doubt, is made more difficult by the present attitude of biological science, which refuses to hear of the inheritance of acquired characters by succeeding generations. (pp. 99–100)

Nonetheless, he insisted with imposing obstinacy on not being able to "do without this factor in biological evolution."

tions they may have become 'organized' as an inherited psychical endowment. Who can decide whether such things as 'innate ideas' exist, or whether in the present instance they have operated, either alone or in conjunction with education, to bring about the permanent fixing of taboos?" One is reminded here of the completely different mode of transmission that Freud discusses in the same work but obviously did not take up again later: "Psycho-analysis has shown us that everyone possesses in his unconscious mental activity an apparatus which enables him to interpret other people's reactions, that is, to undo the distortions which other people have imposed on the expression of their feelings. An unconscious understanding such as this of all the customs, ceremonies and dogmas left behind by the original relation to the father may have made it possible for later generations to take over their heritage of emotion" (p. 159).

36. Although there is no indication of it in Freud's work, it seems improbable that he did not peripherally follow, for instance, the heated discussion concerning the Viennese biologist Paul Kammerer. In the first decades of the century Kammerer had conducted experiments with toads and lizards which, although not intended by him as such, were construed as attempts to prove the inheritance of acquired characteristics and were suspected of having been falsified. Arthur Koestler (1971) gave an account of Kammerer's story. Freud (1919h, p. 238) once benevolently quoted Kammerer's speculative 1919 book, *Das Gesetz der Serie* (The law of series). That the Darwinism-Lamarckism discussion was pursued by Freud's Viennese group of collaborators is verified in part by the reflections of Fritz Wittels (1912, esp. pp. 1–19), mentioned by Freud in his draft.

Why did he refuse to renounce it? He himself indicated a few reasons. Evidently he could not imagine the force—the pathogenic terror—of the threat of castration, the undying, inexorable intensity of the Oedipus complex and the guilt feelings connected with it, operating anew in every generation, as anything but biologically—genetically—determined. Indeed, these feelings were rooted in the "phylogenetic memory-trace . . . from the prehistory of the primal family, when the jealous father actually robbed his son of his genitals if the latter became troublesome to him as a rival with a woman" (1940a [1938], p. 190n). The traumatic real experience in Freud's early conception of the etiology of hysteria appears in fully developed psychoanalytic theory set back into the distant past of the prehistory of the species, that is, transposed from the ontogenetic to the phylogenetic dimension. When viewed from this perspective, the psycho-Lamarckian components of metapsychology are something like a bracket between two stages in the development of Freudian theory. For him to give them up would presumably also have meant to play down psychoanalysis, at least to question its claim to universal validity as a fundamental transcultural statement on the human condition. Furthermore, the postulate helped Freud bridge "the gulf between individual and group psychology." At the same time he hoped to bridge the gulf that "earlier periods of human arrogance had torn too wide apart between mankind and the animals" (1939a [1934–38], p. 100), because he saw in the archaic inheritance of *Homo sapiens* the analogue to the instinctual equipment of animals. And he probably harbored the hope of overcoming yet another gulf, the one between the natural sciences and the humanities (together with the corresponding contradiction in his own academic identity) by means of a metapsychologically, metabiologically supported psychoanalysis.[37]

Freud's obstinacy in still denying any doubts about the existence of a Lamarckian mode of inheritance in the middle to end of the 1930s[38] already shows idiosyncratic traits, even though the revolutionary discoveries of molecular genetics with respect to the structure of the genetic

37. There may have also been compelling unconscious motives for Freud's insistence on the hypothesis of the primal drama in the prehistoric family, but nothing certain can be determined about them. One might speculate endlessly on the possibility that while Freud was working on *Totem and Taboo,* the rift with Jung was in the making, or that during the time of reflection about the twelfth metapsychological paper, in the loneliness brought on by the war, Freud may have felt like the primal father of psychoanalysis, abandoned by his collaborator-sons.

38. This was the time when T. D. Lysenko in the Soviet Union began his efforts to create a scientific basis for Marxist social theory by means of neo-Lamarckian models of inheritance.

substance and the mechanisms of inheritance did not begin until the 1940s. But that does not hold true for his basic evolutionist position at the time of writing his draft of the twelfth metapsychological paper. He shared this stance with many of his collaborators, not only with Sándor Ferenczi, but with Karl Abraham and especially with C. G. Jung, who likewise compared his archetypes to the instincts of animals and considered them to be genetically fixated. Like all these scientists who had been scientifically trained in the last third of the nineteenth and beginning of the twentieth century and who later became active in the investigation of the psyche, Freud stood in a strictly evolutionist scientific tradition. And it was this tradition that had also embraced psychology at the turn of the century.

Freud did, to be sure, expressly point out that in his youth "the theories of Darwin, which were then of topical interest," strongly attracted him (1925d [1924], p. 8). But the extent, impact, and diversity of this evolutionist influence have come more fully to light only in recent times, since the history of science has turned its attention to the early Freud with renewed interest. Following the works of Lucille B. Ritvo, Frank J. Sulloway (1979) has provided the most extensive reconstruction to date of the Lamarckian-Darwinian background[39] that shimmers so noticeably through the hitherto unknown draft of the twelfth metapsychological paper. According to Sulloway, these specific biological roots of psychoanalysis have not yet been sufficiently appreciated, not least because Freud did not constantly refer to them in his works. The reason for this neglect is not that he wanted to disavow a major tie to his intellectual origins, but because at that time people thought evolutionistically—in the broadest sense, Darwinistically—in a similarly unnoticed, matter-of-fact manner, much as we today structure certain spheres of reality according to Freudian categories.

In outlining the historicoscientific context, we must realize that the explanatory concepts of Darwin and Lamarck were not originally considered antagonistic models.[40] While Darwinism was in its ascendancy, the

39. This is still tenable, even if the subsequent criticism of Sulloway's psychobiological reductionism, his socioepistemological conclusions, and his assessment of the originality of Freud's contribution is justified.

40. Ritvo (1972, p. 281) has shown that this juxtaposition is still present in the work of Carl Claus, professor of zoology at the University of Vienna, whose course on Darwinism Freud attended in his second semester (Bernfeld, 1951, p. 216) and who decisively shaped Freud's evolutionist conceptions—as Ritvo demonstrates.

investigations of Jean-Baptiste Lamarck were rediscovered as a significant pioneering achievement on the way to a scientific theory of evolution: the vitalistic idea that the cause of adaptations could be sought in an urge for perfection inherent in the organism, and the conception—prefigured in myth, also in the Bible—that the environment could provoke directed hereditary changes in organisms. Darwin shared the latter view and, like other scientists of his epoch, strove for theoretical concepts on which this mode of inheritance could be based, because he saw in it a complement to the mechanisms of evolution that he himself had postulated: a complement not only to the undirected hereditary variations of organisms, but also to natural selection which, by assuring greater chances of propagation, favors those variants that provide the types of organisms in question with better adaptation under the conditions of life specific to each instance.

Modern evolutionary genetics has confirmed Darwinian theory in its main features. In particular, it has given a comprehensive picture of the microstructure of hereditary variations, through which this variability and along with it the evolutionary capacity of organisms for change is maintained. Natural selection, now as before, ranks as one of the decisive mechanisms of evolution. From the standpoint of today's knowledge, however, the only part of Lamarck's hypothesis that can be maintained is that environmental influences can undoubtedly produce changes in the organism, but these changes are no more than modifications. They change only the phenotype, while the genotype remains untouched by them; thus they are not hereditary.

Despite its stormy development in recent years and decades, the theory of evolution is still considered incomplete. In a paper that describes its present state and emphasizes the need for supplementation, Gerhard Vollmer (1984) maintains that Darwinian mechanisms do not, for instance, explain the origin of the first living beings, of new species, of man, of complex organ systems (like that of the human eye or brain), or of speech and logic. In the meantime, many additional evolutionary factors have been cited, especially to explain such "macroevolutive" processes. A few, representing modern Darwinism, stand today with equal stature next to the classic Darwinian factors.[41] On the other hand, there has been no confirmation of those investigators who still want to fit neo-Lamarckian

41. See for example Vollmer (1984, pp. 288–290), or Remane, Storch, and Welsch (1980, pp. 152–182).

concepts into the existing cracks in the edifice of causal explanation built by evolutionary theory. To be sure, the bitter fanaticism that was still common in Freud's time in the struggle against every neo-Lamarckian intellectual thrust has abated. As long as there is no conclusive proof of a direct influence of the environment on the genome, the assumption that "the genetic equipment of living organisms is supposed to learn from the environment just as the human brain does"[42] should be considered untenable. Hence every form of instruction theory, according to which information from the environment could be directly formulated into the DNA, as it were, is equally untenable. In principle, there is still the possibility that at some time this state of affairs could change somewhat.[43]

What does this mean, not just for the draft of the twelfth metapsychological paper, but for Freud's metapsychology as a whole? For years it has been pointed out again and again that one of the main pillars of that metapsychology, Fechner's constancy principle, does not stand up to more recent scientific knowledge. It has turned out that there is no biological basis for the view that the organism is striving to keep the level of excitation that predominates in it as low as possible, or to shut out altogether the stimuli that impinge on it.[44] Various authors have demonstrated the inhibiting effect of this nineteenth-century psychobiological principle on Freudian metapsychology—that it, for example, has hindered the development of a differentiated clinical affect theory.[45] Freud himself had no illusions about the vagueness and tentativeness of his metapsychologically relevant ideas about energy; he emphasized that "we know nothing of the nature of the excitatory process that takes place in the elements of the psychical systems, and that we do not feel justified in framing any hypothesis on the subject. We are consequently operating all the time with a large unknown factor, which we are obliged to carry over into every new formula" (1920g, pp. 30–31). Similarly striking expressions of skepticism with regard to the psycho-Lamarckian sphere of ideas are absent from the later works especially. Even in the post-Freudian discussion of metapsychology within psychoanalysis, the antiquated elements in Freud's conceptions of evolutionary biology seem not to have

42. Jacob (1982 [1981], p. 15).
43. See for example Weiner (1965, p. 15).
44. See Holt (1965, pp. 108–109).
45. See Modell (1981, p. 393).

been scrutinized in a similarly thorough manner and not, in the light of new knowledge, to have been revised like the physicalistic legacy, the energetic-neuropsychological conceptions.[46]

But not merely specific pieces of theory that catch one's eye in reading the draft of the twelfth metapsychological paper are antiquated. What must appear to the reader as equally out of date, even though the esthetic charm of the second part is closely bound up with it, is the tendency to the grand theoretical scheme, to the forcefully simplifying reconstruction of the evolutionary history of basic features of the *conditio humana*. The phylogenetic development of these basic features, such as speech,[47] is reconstructed in the form of chains of events conceived linearly with respect to time, primal dramas—brilliantly reductionistic ideas, which from the standpoint of today, certainly, are modeled more on myth[48] than on scientific theory.

One could ask pointedly whether the draft overview, with its phylogenetic second part, thus provides an additional argument for dispensing with Freudian metapsychology. Just such a demand, although based on other considerations, has been raised for several years by representatives of various schools—among others hermeneuticists and structuralists, proponents of "action language"—in other words, by those primarily interested in the language aspect of the process of interpretation, in the philosophy of language and linguistics. Hence this demand would lead to establishing psychoanalysis as a humanistic, historical, linguistic, and social science and to declaring Freud's attempt to provide psychoanalysis with a scientific

46. Pribram and Gill (1976), for instance.

47. On the subject of modern means of access to the problem of the evolution of speech, see for instance Schwidetzky (1973).

48. Freud knew, of course, that the transitions between the two are fluid, and he once spoke about the "scientific myth of the father of the primal horde" (1921c, p. 135); in *An Autobiographical Study* (1925d [1924], p. 68), he even called his hypothesis of the murder of the primal father a "vision." The early psychoanalysts were not the only advocates of this type of theory, which at the time was widespread in biological, anthropological, and sociological writings. See for instance the evolutionistically oriented cultural-anthropological authors cited by Freud in the fourth essay of *Totem and Taboo,* whose universalitic theses had of course already come under fire within their own discipline at the time *Totem and Taboo* was being written. See especially Atkinson's constructions (1903) of the primal conditions of human communal life, the "bloody tragedy" (p. 231), the "old-world drama" (p. 232)—namely the sons' murder of the "solitary paternal tyrant" (p. 228)—the role of mother love in setting up the first norms that hold in check the deadly jealousy between fathers and sons and by means of exogamy ensure family cohesion—all of this is reminiscent of the hypothetical line of argumentation in *Totem and Taboo*.

basis an ahistorical "scientistic self-misunderstanding";[49] it would, in effect, pull up the somatic-biological anchor. Insofar as metapsychology has to do with formulating statements of the highest degree of generalization, basically with describing and explaining species-specific characteristics, the discussion must necessarily address biological phenomena—the body.

Certainly our present examination of the context of the draft of the twelfth metapsychological paper is not the place for an appraisal of this discussion. In summarizing it critically, Arnold H. Modell (1981) has pleaded against dispensing with and in favor of revising the metapsychology.[50] Even though central pieces of the content of this metapsychology have become antiquated, its heuristic functions are of undiminished importance and present-day relevance for both the psychoanalytic theoretician and the clinician. Modell subjects these functions to a careful analysis that he summarizes in the statement, "Without metapsychology we cannot begin to think" (p. 395). With that he takes up Freud's late dictum: "Without metapsychological speculation and theorizing—I had almost said 'phantasying'—we shall not get another step forward" (1937c, p. 225).[51]

Years earlier, not long after the draft of his overview of the transference neuroses, Freud in *Beyond the Pleasure Principle* (1920g, p. 60) pondered "our speculation upon the life and death instincts" and ascertained in a manner as free of illusion as it was clairvoyant:

On the other hand it should be made quite clear that the uncertainty of our speculation has been greatly increased by the necessity for borrowing from the science of biology. Biology is truly a land of unlimited possibilities. We may expect it to give us the most surprising information and we cannot guess what answers it will return in a few dozen years to the questions we have put to it. They

49. Habermas (1972 [1968], pp. 246–273).

50. See Holt (1981) for a comprehensive presentation, in which the significance of the system-theoretical approach to a revision of the metapsychology is raised.

51. This is the famous place where Freud, a sentence earlier, speaks of the "Witch Metapsychology" in connection with the quotation from *Faust,* "We must call the Witch to our help after all!" One suspects that this metaphor, ironically, is also haunted by the witch Cañizares from the "Dogs' Colloquy" by Cervantes (1972 [1613], pp. 195–252). In that dialogue from the *Exemplary Stories,* the dog Berganza reports on how the witch entertained him with a lecture on a comprehensive theology based on pairs of opposites (sin/morality, sensuality/abstemiousness, reality/fantasy). Metapsychology is likewise exquisitely dualistically constructed. Furthermore, Freud and his boyhood friend Eduard Silberstein had in their high school days playfully identified with the two talking dogs. (Freud's letters to Silberstein are currently being prepared for publication.)

may be of a kind which will blow away the whole of our artificial structure of hypotheses.

No one will dispute that in the intervening decades biology has, in fact, proved to be "a land of unlimited possibilities," not only because of the revolutionary innovations in molecular biology and genetics, but also with regard to developments in the field of epistemology.[52] Everywhere one observes the beginnings of a new kind of theoretical interweaving of psyche and soma,[53] which seem to make possible a gradual transcendence of the traditional Cartesian schisms of body/soul, brain/mind, natural sciences/humanities, as well as an easing of the subject/object dichotomy.

Only if the metapsychological claim and along with it the connection to biology are maintained within psychoanalysis can psychoanalysts stay alert to these developments and prevent an encapsulation of the Freudian legacy from the discourse of the neighboring disciplines. Even if only a few are able to take active part in such investigations, it is conceivable that good questions, particularly those that bring the dimension of the unconscious to the fore, could be put by psychoanalysts to the representatives of other disciplines. These questions would be derived from the mode of understanding peculiar to the psychoanalytic situation—that oscillation between experiential, empathic intersubjectivity and observing-reflecting objectivity which characterizes the psychoanalytic method that is independent of obsolete metapsychological pieces of theory. At the same time, it would mean handing down Freud's then completely new epistemological position between the natural and the humanistic sciences. For he was radical in two directions: in the impetus of his analysis of civilization, critical of society and religion, and in his relentless insistence on the final anchoring of all human behavior in the pleasure-creating, mortal biological-organic substrate.[54] To deprive psychoanalysis of its metapsychological dimension

52. Two publications should be mentioned as illustrations: Jean Piaget's *Biology and Knowledge: An Essay on the Relations Between Organic Regulations and Cognitive Processes* (1971) and the work of Humberto Maturana (1982) on biological epistemology, in which Maturana goes beyond the traditional man-machine models and constructs a new theory of living systems and of the biologically based subject dependency of the process of knowledge.

53. As two examples see the writings on the biogram (1973) of the anthropologist and zoologist Earl W. Count, and Thure von Uexküll's search for a paradigm of psychosomatic medicine to operate with the concepts of situational circle (*Situationskreis*), time configuration (*Zeitgestalt*), individual reality, program, system, and sign (1979, chaps. 1 to 5, in collaboration with W. Wesiack; 1980, pp. 63 ff.).

54. It is certainly no coincidence that among Freud's collaborators progressive spirits like

would mean, from the standpoint of the theory of knowledge, a step backward from Freud's revolutionary intellectual thrust, a new revisionism. Apart from that, it would then be difficult to gain access to an understanding of human phenomena related to those psychical, or psychophysical, processes of structure formation that are earliest ontogenetically and that arise from the organic matrix.

Back to the draft of the twelfth metapsychological paper. Let me emphasize one last time that Freud, for well-considered reasons, did *not* allow the fair copy to be published. A number of reasons can be given for the fact that the draft is nevertheless now being published contrary to its author's intention (like another foundered document, the fundamental "Project for a Scientific Psychology" of 1895, which was rediscovered along with the letters to Wilhelm Fliess).

The text and the discussion with Sándor Ferenczi reconstructed from the correspondence convey to us a rare direct impression of the ingenuousness, the playful factor, in Freud's creative process. They underscore the significance of imagination in scientific creativity overall—perhaps precisely *because* Freud did not let the result stand at the end, *because* his "daringly playful fantasy," after he had let loose the reins, was subsequently hauled in and overpowered by his "relentlessly realistic criticism," a movement that, incidentally, is foreshadowed in the final paragraph of the draft. Lightness, childlike-youthful curiosity, and the ability to be surprised, to be enthusiastic, a friendly letting-each-other-matter, the unconditionally fact-oriented reciprocal stimulating and mutually correcting—in short, the human and dialogic culture that is a hallmark of this phase of the Freud-Ferenczi friendship—may well serve as a model of scientific collaboration.

Inasmuch as it brings its neo-Lamarckian elements to the fore in a particularly extreme and forceful manner, the draft could give rise to a productive critique of metapsychology, one that does not play down the importance of these problematic pieces and furthers a modernization of theory.[55]

Sándor Ferenczi and Siegfried Bernfeld understood this double radicality and tried to continue it in their own works, even though Ferenczi's bioanalytic studies and Bernfeld's libidometric experiments may have remained speculative or gone completely astray because they lacked a suitable conceptual apparatus.

55. An attempt of this sort was made many years ago in the United States at an interdisciplinary conference (Greenfield and Lewis, 1965).

Of the seven rejected metapsychological papers the twelfth evidently assumed a special place in Freud's estimation. Its second part fascinated him; for he does not expand as fully or as committedly on any other passage of the seven lost texts in the letters that have been preserved from the war years. Certainly, some of the answers attempted in the draft may not be quite convincing to us today. Still, the relevance of some of the questions that Freud did not again take up in this form remains undiminished. One example is consideration of whether what strikes us today as pathological and life inhibiting in the inner world of the neurotic and psychotic could have been an adaptive reaction of the species, necessary for its survival, to threatening changes in the external conditions of life and traumatic events in its evolutionary beginnings. Thus, the draft should not be read merely as a historical curiosity.

In the face of our modern doubts about a Lamarckian mode of inheritance and in view of our changed, pluralistic way of theorizing, Havelock Ellis' observation in his early critique (1910, p. 523) of Freud's Leonardo study (1910c) seems to apply equally well to the hitherto unknown draft of the twelfth metapsychological paper, with its many individual insights still to be uncovered. Ellis was of the opinion that even if Freud does now and then use a very thin thread for his hypotheses, he hardly ever fails to string pearls with it—and they retain their value regardless of whether the thread holds or breaks.

References

Unless otherwise indicated, citations of Freud's works in the text are to *The Standard Edition of the Complete Psychological Works of Sigmund Freud,* 24 vols., edited by James Strachey (London: Hogarth Press, 1953–74), here abbreviated *S.E.* The German citations are to the *Gesammelte Werke,* 18 vols., edited by Anna Freud, with the collaboration of M. Bonaparte, E. Bibring, W. Hoffer, E. Kris, and O. Isakower (Frankfurt: Fischer Verlag, 1940–52, 1968), and to the *Sigmund Freud Studienausgabe,* 11 vols., edited by A. Mitscherlich, A. Richards, and J. Strachey, with a supplementary volume edited by Ilse Grubrich-Simitis (Frankfurt: Fischer Verlag, 1969–75). Works in the *Standard Edition,* some of which have letters after the dates, are cited in conformity with the Alan Tyson–James Strachey "Chronological Hand-List of Freud's Works" in the *International Journal of Psycho-Analysis* (1956), 37:19–33, and the 1975 volume *Sigmund Freud Konkordanz und Gesamtbibliographie,* which accompanies the *Studienausgabe.* Dates when the works were written, where these are known, are enclosed in square brackets after the dates of publication. Dates of original publication of English translations of works by other authors are also enclosed in square brackets.

Atkinson, J. J. 1903. "Primal Law." In J. J. Atkinson and A. Lang, *Social Origins and Primal Law,* pp. 209–294. London: Longmans.

Balint, M. 1930. "Psychosexual Parallels to the Fundamental Law of Biogenetics." In *Primary Love and Psychoanalytic Technique,* pp. 11–41. New York: Liveright, 1953; London: Hogarth Press, 1952.

Bernfeld, S. 1951. "Sigmund Freud, M.D., 1882–1885." *International Journal of Psycho-Analysis,* 32:204–217.

Bettelheim, B. 1983. *Freud and Man's Soul.* New York: Knopf.

Cervantes, M. de. 1972 [1613]. *Exemplary Stories.* Trans. C. A. Jones. Baltimore: Penguin Books.

Count, E. W. 1973. *Being and Becoming Human: Essays on the Biogram.* New York: Van Nostrand.

Darwin, C. 1871. *The Descent of Man.* 2 vols. London: John Murray.

Ellis, H. 1910. "Review (under the Rubric 'Epitome of Current Literature') of Sigmund Freud's *A Psycho-analytic Study of Leonardo da Vinci.*" *Journal of Mental Science,* 56:522–523.

Ferenczi, S. 1913. "Stages in the Development of the Sense of Reality." In *Sex in Psychoanalysis.* New York: Basic Books, 1950. Also in *First Contributions to Psycho-Analysis,* pp. 213–239. Trans. E. Jones. London: Hogarth Press, 1952.

——— 1968 [1924]. "Thalassa: A Theory of Genitality." Trans. H. A. Bunker. New York: Norton.

Freud, S. 1900a. *The Interpretation of Dreams. S.E.* 4, 5.

——— 1901b. *The Psychopathology of Everyday Life. S.E.* 6.

——— 1905d. *Three Essays on the Theory of Sexuality. S.E.* 7:125–245.

——— 1910c. *Leonardo da Vinci and a Memory of His Childhood. S.E.* 11:59–137.

——— 1911b. "Formulations on the Two Principles of Mental Functioning." *S.E.* 12:215–226.

——— 1912–13. *Totem and Taboo. S.E.* 13:1–162.

——— 1913i. "The Disposition to Obsessional Neurosis." *S.E.* 12:313–326.

——— 1914c. "On Narcissism: An Introduction." *S.E.* 14:69–102.

——— 1914d. "On the History of the Psycho-Analytic Movement." *S.E.* 14: 3–66.

——— 1915c. "Instincts and Their Vicissitudes." *S.E.* 14:111–140.

——— 1915d. "Repression." *S.E.* 14:143–158.

——— 1915e. "The Unconscious." *S.E.* 14:161–215.

——— 1916–17 [1915–17]. *Introductory Lectures on Psycho-Analysis. S.E.* 15, 16.

——— 1917d [1915]. "A Metapsychological Supplement to the Theory of Dreams." *S.E.* 14:219–235.

——— 1917e [1915]. "Mourning and Melancholia." *S.E.* 14:239–260.

——— 1918b [1914]. "From the History of an Infantile Neurosis." *S.E.* 17:3–123.

——— 1919e. "A Child Is Being Beaten." *S.E.* 17:177–204.

——— 1919h. "The Uncanny." *S.E.* 17:218–256.

——— 1920g. *Beyond the Pleasure Principle. S.E.* 18:3–64.

——— 1921c. *Group Psychology and the Analysis of the Ego. S.E.* 18:67–143.

——— 1923b. *The Ego and the Id. S.E.* 19:3–66.

——— 1925d [1924]. *An Autobiographical Study. S.E.* 20:3–74.

——— 1925j. "Some Psychical Consequences of the Anatomical Distinction between the Sexes." *S.E.* 19:243–258.

——— 1926d [1925]. *Inhibitions, Symptoms and Anxiety. S.E.* 20:77–175.

——— 1926e. *The Question of Lay Analysis. S.E.* 20:179–258.

——— 1930a [1929]. *Civilization and Its Discontents. S.E.* 21:59–145.

——— 1933a [1932]. *New Introductory Lectures on Psycho-Analysis. S.E.* 22:3–182.

——— 1933c. "Sándor Ferenczi," an obituary. *S.E.* 22:226–229.

——— 1937c. "Analysis Terminable and Interminable." *S.E.* 23:211–253.

——— 1939a [1934–38]. *Moses and Monotheism. S.E.* 23:3–137.

——— 1940a [1938]. *An Outline of Psycho-Analysis. S.E.* 23:141–207.

——— 1950a [1895]. "Project for a Scientific Psychology." In *The Origins of Psycho-Analysis,* ed. M. Bonaparte, A. Freud, and E. Kris, pp. 347–445. Trans. E. Mosbacher and J. Strachey. New York: Basic Books, 1954.

——— 1960a. *Letters of Sigmund Freud, 1873–1939,* ed. E. L. Freud. Trans. T. Stern and J. Stern. New York: Basic Books.

——— 1965a. A *Psycho-Analytic Dialogue: The Letters of Sigmund Freud and Karl Abraham,* ed. H. C. Abraham and E. L. Freud. New York: Basic Books; London: Hogarth Press.

——— 1966a [1912–36]. *Sigmund Freud and Lou Andreas-Salomé Letters,* ed. E. Pfeiffer. New York: Harcourt Brace Jovanovich, 1972; London: Hogarth Press, 1972.

——— 1971a [1909–16]. *James Jackson Putnam and Psychoanalysis: Letters between Putnam and Sigmund Freud, Ernest Jones, William James, Sándor Ferenczi, and Morton Prince, 1877–1917,* ed. N. G. Hale, Jr. Cambridge, Massachusetts: Harvard University Press.

——— 1985. *The Complete Letters of Sigmund Freud to Wilhelm Fliess, 1887–1904,* ed. J. M. Masson. Cambridge, Massachusetts: Belknap Press, Harvard University Press.

Greenfield, N. S., and Lewis, W. C., eds. 1965. *Psychoanalysis and Current Biological Thought.* Madison: University of Wisconsin Press.

Grubrich-Simitis, I. 1977. "Notizen zum Manuskript." In Sigmund Freud, *Das Motiv der Kästchenwahl: Faksimileausgabe,* ed. I. Grubrich-Simitis, pp. 39–46. Frankfurt am Main: S. Fischer Verlag.

Habermas, J. 1972 [1968]. *Knowledge and Human Interests.* Trans. J. J. Shapiro. Boston: Beacon Press.

Holt, R. R. 1965. "A Review of Some of Freud's Biological Assumptions and Their Influence on His Theories." In Greenfield and Lewis, 1965, pp. 93–124.

——— 1981. "The Death and Transfiguration of Metapsychology." *International Review of Psycho-Analysis,* 8:129–143.

Jacob, F. 1982 [1981]. *The Possible and the Actual.* Seattle: University of Washington Press.

Jones, E. 1924. Preface to "Glossary for the Use of Translators of Psycho-analytic Works." *International Journal of Psycho-Analysis,* suppl. 1.

——— 1955. *Sigmund Freud: Life and Work,* vol. 2. New York: Basic Books.

——— 1957. *Sigmund Freud: Life and Work,* vol. 3. New York: Basic Books.

Kammerer, P. 1919. *Das Gesetz der Serie: Eine Lehre von den Wiederholungen im Lebens- und Weltgeschehen.* Stuttgart: Deutsche Verlagsanstalt.

Khan, M. R. 1983 [1974]. "Grudge and the Hysteric." In *Hidden Selves: Between Theory and Practice in Psychoanalysis,* pp. 51–58. London: Hogarth Press.

Klein, G. S. 1976. *Psychoanalytic Theory: An Exploration of Essentials.* New York: International Universities Press.

Koestler, A. 1971. *The Case of the Midwife Toad: Work and Theories of the Viennese Biologist Paul Kammerer.* London: Hutchinson.

Kris, A. 1982. *Free Association.* New Haven: Yale University Press.

——— 1984. "The Conflicts of Ambivalence." *Psychoanalytic Study of the Child,* 39:213–234.

Lamarck, J. B. 1963 [1809]. *Zoological Philosophy: An Exposition with Regard to the Natural History of Animals.* New York: Hafner.

Mahoney, P. 1982. *Freud as a Writer.* New York: International Universities Press.

——— 1984. "Further Reflections on Freud and His Writing." *Journal of the American Psychoanalytic Association,* 32:847–864.

Maturana, H. R. 1982. *Erkennen: Die Organisation und Verkörperung von Wirklichkeit, Ausgewählte Arbeiten zur biologischen Epistemologie.* Braunschweig, Wiesbaden: Vieweg.

Modell, A. H. 1981. "Does Metapsychology Still Exist?" *International Journal of Psycho-Analysis,* 62:391–401.

——— 1984. *Psychoanalysis in a New Context.* New York: International Universities Press.

Nagera, H., ed. 1970. *Basic Psychoanalytic Concepts on Metapsychology, Conflicts, Anxiety, and Other Subjects.* Hampstead Clinic Psychoanalytic Library, vol. 4. New York: Basic Books; London: George Allen & Unwin.

Ornston, D. 1982. "Strachey's Influence." *International Journal of Psycho-Analysis,* 63:409–426.

——— 1985. "Freud's Conception Is Different from Strachey's." *Journal of the American Psychoanalytic Association,* 33:379–412.

Paniagua, C. 1982. "Metaphors and Isomorphisms: Analogical Reasoning in *Beyond the Pleasure Principle,*" *Journal of the American Psychoanalytic Association,* 30:509–523.

Piaget, J. 1971. *Biology and Knowledge: An Essay on the Relations between Organic Regulations and Cognitive Processes.* Chicago: University of Chicago Press.

Pines, M. 1985. Guest editorial. *International Journal of Psycho-Analysis,* 66:1–2.

Pribram, K. H., and Gill, M. M. 1976. *Freud's "Project" Reassessed: Preface to Contemporary Cognitive Theory and Neuropsychology.* New York: Basic Books; London: Hutchinson.

Remane, A., Storch, V., and Welsch, U. 1980. *Evolution; Tatsachen und Probleme der Abstammungslehre,* 5th ed. Munich: Deutscher Taschenbuch Verlag (1st ed., 1973).

Ritvo, L. B. 1972. "Carl Claus as Freud's Professor of the New Darwinian Biology." *International Journal of Psycho-Analysis,* 53:277–283.

Sandler, J. 1960. "The Background of Safety." *International Journal of Psycho-Analysis,* 41:352–356.

Schwidetzky, I., ed. 1973. *Über die Evolution der Sprache; Anatomie-Verhaltensforschung-Sprachwissenschaft-Anthropologie, Conditio Humana* Series. Frankfurt am Main: S. Fischer Verlag.

Shafer, R. 1983. *The Analytic Attitude.* New York: Basic Books.

Strachey, A. 1943. *A New German-English Psycho-Analytical Vocabulary.* London: Bailliere, Tindall and Cox.

Strachey, J. 1957a. Editor's introduction to "Papers on Metapsychology." *S.E.* 14:105–107.

——— 1957b. Editor's note to "The Unconscious." *S.E.* 14:161–165.

——— 1959. Editor's introduction to *Inhibitions, Symptoms and Anxiety. S.E.* 20:77–86.

Sulloway, F. J. 1979. *Freud, Biologist of the Mind: Beyond the Psychoanalytic Legend.* New York: Basic Books.

Uexküll, Th. von, ed. 1979. *Lehrbuch der Psychosomatischen Medizin.* Munich: Urban & Schwarzenberg.

——— 1980. "Das Problem der Entsprechung von Rollen und Gegenrollen bei Arzt und Patient." In *Zur Psychoanalyse der Objektbeziehungen,* ed. G. Jappe and C. Nedelmann, pp. 37–73. Stuttgart/Bad Cannstatt: Frommann-Holzboog.

Vollmer, G. 1984. "Die Unvollständigkeit der Evolutionstheorie." In *Moderne Naturphilosophie,* ed. B. Kanitscheider, pp. 285–316. Würzburg: Königshausen und Neumann.

Wallace, E. R. 1983. *Freud and Anthropology: A History and Reappraisal. Psychological Issues* series, monograph 55. New York: International Universities Press.

Weiner, H. 1965. "Psychoanalysis as a Biological Science." In Greenfield and Lewis, 1965, pp. 11–33.

Wittels, F. 1912. *Alles um Liebe; Eine Urweltdichtung.* Berlin: E. Fleischl.